YOGA

for
ATHLETES

Ryanne Cunningham

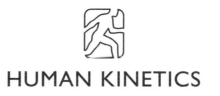

HUMAN KINETICS

Library of Congress Cataloging-in-Publication Data

Names: Cunningham, Ryanne.
Title: Yoga for athletes / Ryanne Cunningham.
Description: Champaign, IL : Human Kinetics, [2017]
Identifiers: LCCN 2016029964 (print) | LCCN 2016032234 (ebook) | ISBN
    9781492522614 (print) | ISBN 9781492531364 (ebook)
Subjects: LCSH: Hatha yoga. | Athletes--Health and hygiene.
Classification: LCC RA781.7 C855 2017 (print) | LCC RA781.7 (ebook) | DDC
    613.7/046--dc23
LC record available at https://lccn.loc.gov/2016029964

ISBN: 978-1-4925-2261-4 (print)

This publication is written and published to provide accurate and authoritative information relevant to the subject matter presented. It is published and sold with the understanding that the author and publisher are not engaged in rendering legal, medical, or other professional services by reason of their authorship or publication of this work. If medical or other expert assistance is required, the services of a competent professional person should be sought.

The web addresses cited in this text were current as of July 2016, unless otherwise noted.

Acquisitions Editor: Michelle Maloney; **Senior Developmental Editor:** Cynthia McEntire; **Senior Managing Editor:** Elizabeth Evans; **Managing Editor:** Caitlin Husted; **Copyeditor:** Joanna Hatzopoulos Portman; **Senior Graphic Designer:** Keri Evans; **Graphic Designer:** Julie L. Denzer; **Cover Designer:** Keith Blomberg; **Photograph (cover):** Neil Bernstein, © Human Kinetics; **Photographs (interior):** Neil Bernstein, © Human Kinetics; **Visual Production Assistant:** Joyce Brumfield; **Photo Production Manager:** Jason Allen; **Senior Art Manager:** Kelly Hendren; **Illustrations:** © Human Kinetics, unless otherwise noted; **Printer:** Versa Press

We thank the Flow Yoga Studio in De Pere, Wisconsin, for assistance in providing the location for the photo shoot for this book.

Human Kinetics books are available at special discounts for bulk purchase. Special editions or book excerpts can also be created to specification. For details, contact the Special Sales Manager at Human Kinetics.

Printed in the United States of America   10 9 8 7 6 5 4 3 2 1

The paper in this book is certified under a sustainable forestry program.

Human Kinetics
Website: www.HumanKinetics.com

United States: Human Kinetics
P.O. Box 5076
Champaign, IL 61825-5076
800-747-4457
e-mail: info@hkusa.com

Canada: Human Kinetics
475 Devonshire Road Unit 100
Windsor, ON N8Y 2L5
800-465-7301 (in Canada only)
e-mail: info@hkcanada.com

Europe: Human Kinetics
107 Bradford Road
Stanningley
Leeds LS28 6AT, United Kingdom
+44 (0) 113 255 5665
e-mail: hk@hkeurope.com

Australia: Human Kinetics
57A Price Avenue
Lower Mitcham,
South Australia 5062
08 8372 0999
e-mail: info@hkaustralia.com

New Zealand: Human Kinetics
P.O. Box 80
Mitcham Shopping Centre,
South Australia 5062
0800 222 062
e-mail: info@hknewzealand.com

E6711

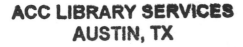

YOGA

for

ATHLETES

CONTENTS

Part II   Poses for Sport-Specific Performance

POSE FINDER

ACKNOWLEDGMENTS

A huge thank-you to my amazing editors and the whole crew who helped me through this process of writing and publishing my first book. All of you have made my dreams come true: Michelle Maloney, Cynthia McEntire, Liz Evans, Sue Outlaw, Neil Bernstein, and the many more whom I did not get the chance to meet.

Tremendous thanks and respect go to the most dedicated, motivated, humble, and inspiring professional athletes I had the honor to teach yoga to through the years. The hours each of you dedicated to yoga practice in your off time and the time you took away from your families to stay healthy for game day are beyond words. I thank each of your families for understanding and pushing you to go to yoga. Most important, I thank each of you for your trust, respect, and humility in allowing me to be your yoga instructor. You made my dreams come true and are beyond friends. Namaste to each of you: Tramon Williams, Jarrett Bush, Randall Cobb, BJ Raji, Sam Barrington, Andy Mulumba, Mike Neal, Micah Hyde, Datone Jones, Damarious Randall, Quinten Rollins, Nathan Palmer, DJ Williams, Greg Jennings, Brandon Bostick, Jermichael Finley, Jerel Worthy, Keifer Sykes, and those whose names cannot be mentioned at this time.

Thanks to talented and inspiring author Joyce Salisbury. I appreciate all the time, energy, and help you gave me in the very beginning of this book to get the ball rolling. I do not know what I would have done without you! You gave me the advice and confidence I needed to be an author. Your knowledge and experience as an author are so inspiring, and I'm so happy to have you as a student, friend, and teacher.

I believe in life there are many reasons why we meet and become friends with others. Thank you, Bradley Berndt, for your friendship, your inspiring positivity, and an introduction to Mindy. Mindy Bennett, you of course have been an inspiration to me through your yoga practice and drive for fitness. I will always thank you for all that you have done for me.

The moment you walked through my studio door, Tyler Dunne, you changed my world. You are an inspiring writer. Because of your talent for writing, you made my dreams come true by being in nationally known yoga magazines that then led to the creation of this book. You have a great presence, and I loved our conversations on sports and fitness. I will always admire your passion for writing and sports.

I can't adequately thank my amazing models who are also my talented, athletic, and fun friends. All of you have made this book so real and inspiring: Abby Widmer, Kevin Dart, Brian Danzinger, and Brennan Hutjens. And to my teachers and models at Flow Yoga Studio: Elisabeth Herbner and David Konshak.

Without the love and support from all my students, Flow Yoga Studio would not exist. Thanks to all of you! I love seeing each of you weekly, and I enjoy watching each of your yoga journeys blossom.

I am grateful to the most inspiring, smart, talented, and down-to-earth teachers in my life: Gwen Lawrence, Liz Arch, and Yancy Scot Schwartz. Because of you three, I have taken my yoga practice to new levels. I learn more each time I see you. I will always continue to admire and learn from the three of you as long as you let me. With so much love and respect to each of you, thanks so much for allowing me to be in your lives and for being such great friends. Namaste.

The friends in my life are always what keep me smiling and feeling alive. Thanks to each of you! From my besties, yoga group, Instagram handstand crew, bunco group, book club, traveling girlfriends, and long-time friends for just being there for me, supporting me, and loving me no matter what. Love you guys!

To my whole family, thank you for believing in me, allowing me to follow my dreams, encouraging me to keep going, and always having my back. All of you are always there for me and you are my heart and soul. Mom, Aunt Kathy, Uncle Gary, Kari, Grant, Gavin, and Grady, thank you for your love.

Mom, thank you for all of your hard work as a single mother. Because of you, I am the woman I am today. You have always pushed me to follow my heart and dreams, and you always believed in me. I love you for that, Mom. Thank you.

To my cat Gracie. You snuggled next to me, on me, on my computer, even worked your way up into my face through every word in this book . . . except for this acknowledgment. My baby Gracie passed two days before I wrote this part. You, baby girl, showed me what love really is: simplicity in life and just being. I miss you and love you, princess.

And a big thank-you to my love, Brad, for the support, belief, and kindness you showed me during this journey. Thank you for being my best friend, being you, and just being there when I needed you most. I could not have done this book without you! You are a great person, and I love you for that.

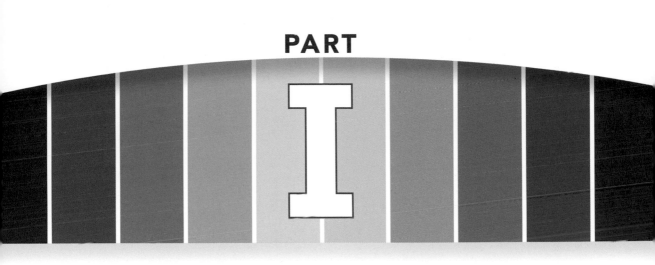

PART

I

Athletic Benefits of Yoga

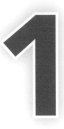

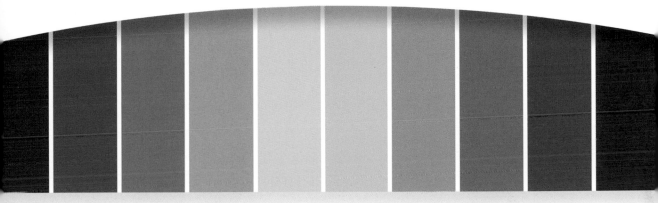

WHY DO YOGA?

Athletes—especially professional athletes—have trainers who prepare weight training regimens and stretching exercises for them. Athletes have coaches who observe and correct every movement they perform, and they have physicians who check them for injuries. So, do they really need one more way to train? The answer is yes. They should do yoga, because it provides an extra edge through balance, flexibility, breath, and mental sharpness.

The desire to improve is a key component of competitive sport, and all athletes have room for improvement in their sport or training. Athletic careers are characterized by a chase for a better time, a stronger body, better split-second decisions, the ability to take a harder hit, and other ways of advancing. Every small improvement gives athletes an edge in achieving their goals for better performance. Whether they are professional athletes competing against others or amateurs competing to improve themselves, yoga can bring that special edge to their performance.

Training for your specific sport or activity includes strengthening and conditioning your muscles. Each sport emphasizes some muscle groups over others. Yoga can help bring balance to all the muscle groups of the body. This text isn't as comprehensive as an anatomy text, but it does address the major muscle groups that are targeted in the exercises. Figure

1.1 provides an overview of the major muscle groups from the anterior (front) and posterior (rear) view. Refer back to this figure as you learn the exercises in this book.

Yoga is a particularly effective training tool for athletes because it weaves together stretching, strength building, breathing, and balance. This combination offers an edge. Each athlete has unique needs, and a yoga practice benefits everyone in a special way. This chapter outlines some of the many ways that a yoga practice can improve athletic performance. For each of the benefits of yoga for athletic performance, you can find yoga poses to maximize that benefit.

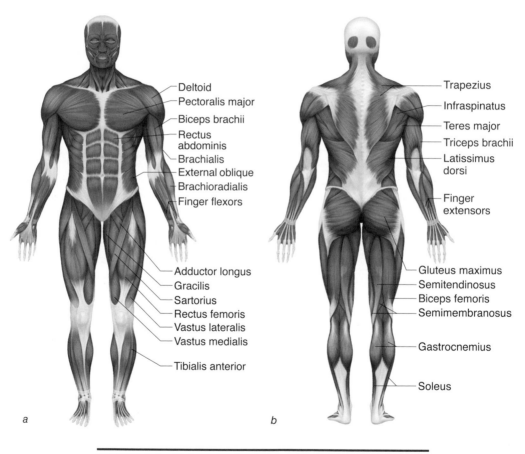

FIGURE 1.1   Major muscle groups: *(a)* anterior; *(b)* posterior.

Aid in Muscle Recovery

Athletes need rest time between workouts to allow muscles to recover. Coaches spend a lot of time and research trying to determine the optimal rest time necessary before a game or competition. Muscles have to be ready to go, but if they are too rested they will not perform optimally. What causes the muscle fatigue that sets in when the body is in constant motion?

As you work out, your muscles use the oxygen you take in, burning it to create energy. The deep breathing in yoga helps bring this much-needed oxygen to the muscles. As muscles contract, they produce by-products of this metabolism, and the most common is lactic acid. As the lactic acid and other by-products of the muscle metabolism build up, muscle fatigue sets in, and the body can no longer perform to its maximum capacity. Rest and drinking lots of water are recommended to clear the waste products from the muscles so that they can contract to their maximum capacity again. The critical question that trainers and coaches know all too well is what is the optimal rest time to clear the muscles? If you wait too long, you lose valuable training time; if you don't wait long enough, you risk injury. The problem is compounded by the fact that everyone is different; one size does not fit all. Each person has to find the perfect formula for maximum and rapid recovery, and yoga can help.

The goal of recovery is to clear the muscles of waste products, including lactic acid, to allow the fibers to fire again. Hydration helps by flushing waste products out of the body, but proper stretching of muscles will also more rapidly restore function. Yoga practitioners have always known the best way to stretch.

When muscles become tight after exercise, you need to stretch them out, but you have to do it correctly. You have to be sure to focus your stretching on the muscle, not the tendon. With proper stretching, the muscle improves its elasticity so that it doesn't tighten up during exercise. The main goal is to hold the stretch for a long period of time (10 to 20 breaths); a shorter stretch is not as effective. While holding the stretch, maintain a constant deep breath to get the blood supply to the muscle being stretched. This deep breathing helps to bring nutrients to the muscle for energy to help with muscle recovery and to recharge the muscle for your next explosive workout. Chapter 2 discusses yoga techniques for breathing, and stretches for restoring your muscles after a workout are included throughout the book. The more quickly your muscles bounce back, the sooner you can get back to training so that you will gain a competitive edge.

Sometimes after workouts, the legs feel heavy and fatigued. The best thing you can do for these tired legs is elevate them to improve circulation and let the fluids drain back into the lymphatic system. A great technique is legs up the wall pose. Like all yoga poses, this one has multiple benefits. It helps your muscles bounce back while providing other benefits, such as improving digestion, reenergizing the body, and quieting the mind.

Legs Up the Wall Pose

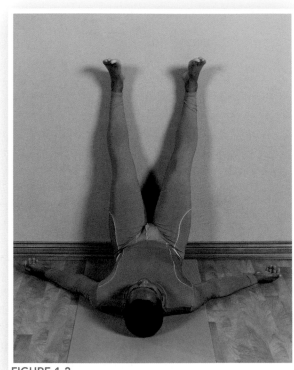

FIGURE 1.2

Muscles

Hamstrings

1. Face a wall.
2. Lie on your back, and put your legs straight up the wall (figure 1.2).
3. Your hips can either touch the wall or be a few inches away from the wall.
4. Relax your arms by your sides with your palms facing up.
5. Relax in the pose for at least 5 minutes; 10 to 15 minutes is better.

Modifications

If your hamstrings are tight, lie on your back with your hips a few inches away from the wall and your legs up the wall with both knees bent. Plant your feet on the wall. For tight hamstrings, add a yoga block or blanket under your hips to elevate them.

Prevent Injuries

Professional and amateur athletes alike worry about injuries that will interfere with their sport. For many athletes, a season-ending injury is their greatest concern. What causes most sports injuries? Leaving aside accidents, which can and do happen, most sports injuries come from these five main causes:

1. Lack of a careful warm-up
2. Quick motions and twisting motions that stress joints
3. Imbalance that trains one part of the body over others
4. Tightness of highly-trained muscles that lose flexibility
5. Overuse of the muscles

Yoga practice can help prevent injuries from the first four causes. Yoga poses emphasize strengthening, stretching, and balance among all parts of the body. A yoga practice begins with a warm-up that prepares all the muscles and connective tissues for vigorous exercise. Then, yoga postures make sure that muscles surrounding vulnerable joints such as knees and ankles are strong enough to allow for the quick, explosive movements that mark athletic performance. As you work through this book, you will notice that even small, usually neglected muscles are noted.

Imbalanced training is a serious problem in many sports. Some sports, such as tennis, golf, and baseball pitching, use one side of the body more than the other. This imbalance adds stress on joints and can easily lead to injury on both the weaker and stronger sides. Some sports have particular stress on one body part. For example, cyclists often experience neck pain from leaning over the handlebars for extended periods. The neck compensates so that the rider can see forward. Sometimes the pressure of the body weight leaning forward on the arms can cause pain in the upper back and neck. A yoga practice can bring the parts of the body back into balance, reducing the probability of injures.

Finally and most importantly, yoga can restore and preserve the flexibility that is often sacrificed by strength-building exercises. Muscle tightness may lead to torn muscles and a season-ending injury. Yoga's emphasis on stretching muscles will lengthen them, reducing the potential for injury and allowing the connective tissue to be restored. A regular yoga and stretch routine keeps an athlete's muscles loose and flexible so that instead of a torn muscle during a game, an athlete may only slightly pull a muscle. Instead of a season-ending injury, an athlete can reduce the number of games missed thanks to flexibility. Each sport requires different stretches to complement the trained muscles. See part II to learn how to tailor your yoga practice to your sport.

All athletes want to perform to the best of their ability, and in doing so they often run the risk of overusing their muscles. Yoga training can bring balance and flexibility to strong muscles to reduce the potential of overuse injuries. Avoiding these injuries is key to improving athletic performance.

The poses throughout this book will help you prevent athletic injuries. Poses are beneficial done on their own or in sequence with other poses. A common sequence of yoga poses is moving from upward-facing dog pose to downward-facing dog pose (or cobra pose to downward-facing dog pose), both of which are described next. These poses accomplish the balanced stretch of all parts of the body, and they are strong poses for building muscles. These poses appear several times throughout this book; refer to the following descriptions as needed.

Upward-Facing Dog Pose

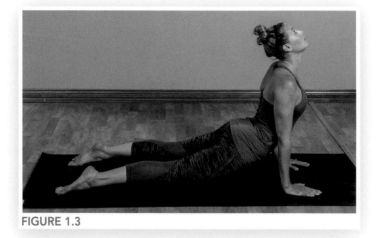

FIGURE 1.3

Muscles

Triceps, infraspinatus and teres minor, rhomboids, trapezius, quadriceps, gluteus maximus

1. Lie facedown with your hands placed on the mat and under your shoulders.
2. Inhale as you lift your chest and straighten your arms.
3. Roll over your toes to the tops of your feet.
4. Engage your quadriceps to lift your knees off the floor, keeping your legs straight (figure 1.3).
5. Keep your shoulders down and back, away from your ears.
6. Pull your shoulder blades toward each other and down your back.
7. Align the shoulders over the wrists.
8. Keep your palms pressing down into your mat, maintaining straight arms.
9. Gaze forward to lengthen and relax your neck.
10. Push your shoulders back as your shoulder blades press down.

11. Press the tops of your feet down into your mat as you engage your quadriceps and lift your knees off the floor, maintaining a slight engagement of your gluteal muscles.

Safety Tip

Keep a slight engagement of your abdominal muscles to prevent discomfort in your low back. If you have any problems in the low back or shoulders, do cobra pose instead.

Cobra Pose

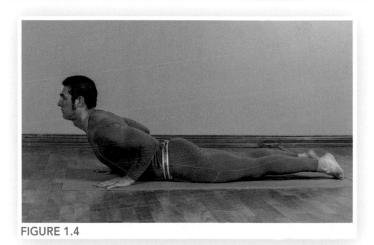

FIGURE 1.4

Muscles

Rectus abdominis, quadriceps, sartorius, pectoralis major, deltoids

1. Lie facedown with your legs extended, your arms down along your sides, and your forehead resting on the mat.
2. Bend your elbows, then plant your hands on the mat next to your rib cage.
3. Lift your forehead off the floor, lengthening your chest forward and upward as you softly press your palms into the mat (figure 1.4).
4. At the same time, stretch your legs as you engage your quadriceps and press the tops of your feet down into the mat.
5. Keep your abdominal muscles engaged, and tuck your tailbone toward your heels while in this pose.

Modification

Lengthen through the legs and hover your legs up from the floor as you pull your chest forward.

Safety Tip

Keep your tailbone tucking toward your heels to prevent sinking into your low back, keep creating length in your spine, and keep your core engaged while in the pose.

Downward-Facing Dog Pose

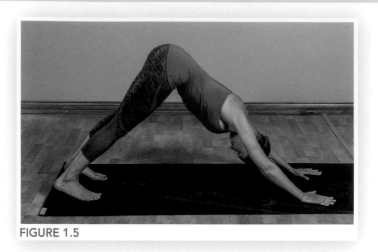

FIGURE 1.5

Muscles

Triceps, infraspinatus, teres minor, rhomboids, trapezius, erector spinae, quadratus lumborum, hamstrings, gastrocnemius and soleus (calf muscles), gluteal muscles

1. Lie facedown with your hands on the mat underneath your shoulders.
2. Exhale as you lift your hips up and back and roll over your toes.
3. Press into your hands to lengthen your arms.
4. Roll your shoulders out away from your ears.
5. Relax your neck.
6. Lengthen your spine as you lift your hips.
7. Press down through your heels, and straighten your legs (figure 1.5).
8. Make sure your hands are shoulder-width apart and your index fingers point to the top of your mat.
9. Separate the fingers wide.

Modification

If your hamstrings are tight and your spine is rounding, bend both knees slightly and tip your pelvis so that the tailbone reaches upward. Focus on a long spine by pressing into your palms and lifting your hips.

Safety Tip

Watch for any hyperextension. In this pose it is easy to hyperextend the elbows and knees.

Reduce Stress, Increase Focus, and Relieve Tension

Working out puts a natural stress on the body, but it is a good stress. Exercise helps you to let go of the stresses of daily life rather than hold on to them. However, when working out is your career or you are serious about a sport to the point where you place high expectations on yourself, exercise can actually create stress instead of alleviating it. Yoga can help athletes work through those stresses. Here's how it works: When you step onto a yoga mat and put your body through a sequence of unfamiliar poses and stretches, it actually helps you to de-stress. The stress hormone cortisol is carried in your body during stressful times. While practicing a yoga sequence, you go through a series of movements, poses, and deep breathing, which decreases your levels of cortisol. Afterward, you feel more relaxed and less stressed.

Another way yoga can help an athlete reduce stress is to require focusing on the pose, which means staying in the present instead of thinking about the past or the future. During yoga practice, at some point a challenging pose is presented. At first you might cringe, not wanting to do the pose. However, once you have worked your way in and out of that pose, you realize that you were so focused on it that you didn't think about anything else. This is yoga; it brings you into the moment and allows you to focus.

A final way yoga can reduce stress and help you practice living in the moment is through concentrated breathing. Yogic breathing is explained in more depth in the next chapter. For now, start by sitting and concentrating on your breath. It takes practice to focus so intently, but it will calm the mind and reduce stress in the body. Seated cross-legged pose is a great pose to practice for a calming, quiet moment or a meditative practice.

Seated Cross-Legged Pose

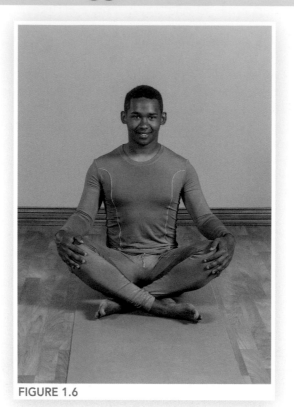

FIGURE 1.6

Muscles

Psoas, quadratus lumborum, erector spinae, rhomboids, latissimus dorsi, rectus abdominis

1. Sit on the floor.
2. Bend both knees, crossing your feet at the ankles.
3. Sit tall, lengthening your spine through the top of your head.
4. Relax your shoulders away from your ears.
5. Place your hands on your knees (figure 1.6).
6. Look forward and sit for 2 to10 minutes.

Modification

If this position is uncomfortable, place a block or blanket under your hips to elevate you for more comfort and to maintain a long spine.

Safety Tip

A common problem in this pose is knee discomfort. To allow space in your knees and hips, slide your feet forward in front of your hips and put the soles of your feet together.

Strengthen Underused Muscles

It's easy to fall into a training routine to strengthen areas that are most important for your sport. In fact, the most serious athletes want to focus on improving the muscles that affect their performance. However, athletes must remember that the body is connected; when you neglect one area of our body, it creates weakness and imbalance. After some time and overuse, imbalances in the body can trigger discomfort in ligaments and joints, which can lead to more serious injuries.

Athletes put their bodies through a lot of movement during practices, and they tend to forget the little areas of the body that actually take most of the weight and do most of the work. Throughout this book you will learn poses that focus on all areas of the body, and especially in chapter 8 you will notice the small muscles. For now, practicing the wrist stretch will remind you of the importance of the small muscles and joints that athletes too often take for granted. This pose will help with the mobility of your wrists not only for yoga but also for sport and training.

Wrist Stretch

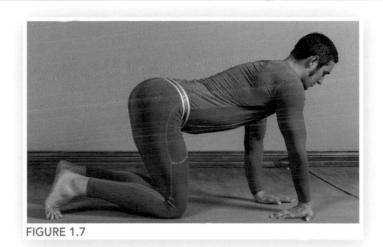

FIGURE 1.7

Muscles

Pronator quadratus, flexor carpi radialis, flexor carpi ulnaris, brachioradialis, palmar brevis, flexor digitorum superficialis

1. Start on your hands and knees.
2. Align your shoulders over your wrists and hips over knees.
3. Turn your right hand clockwise around so that your fingers point to your right knee.
4. Plant your palm down on the mat.
5. Keep your right arm straight and your right shoulder back away from your ear.

(continued)

6. Keep your palm flat on the mat.
7. Shift your hips back slowly toward your heels until you feel a stretch in your lower arm (figure 1.7). Hold this position for 5 to 10 breaths.
8. To come out of the pose, shift your hips forward.
9. Repeat on the left side, turning your left hand counterclockwise.

Modification

Come to seated position on your knees and bring your palms together in prayer, pressing them together. Slowly lower your wrists and lift your elbows up (figure 1.8).

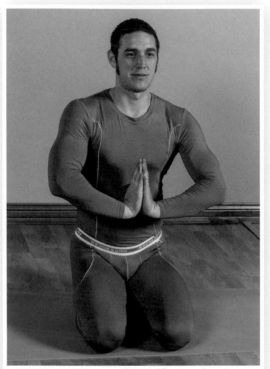

FIGURE 1.8 Wrist stretch modification, hands in prayer position.

Safety Tip

You should feel a good stretch in the wrist, without pain. If you feel pain, you have stretched too far.

Build Your Core

Personal trainers and coaches in all sports include core exercises as part of training. Yoga has always emphasized the central muscles that are the foundation of the entire trunk. Core muscles include more than the front abdominal muscles that people refer to as a six-pack. The core muscles also include the low back, muscles surrounding the hip, and the whole area that supports your spine, which are all shown in figure 1.9.

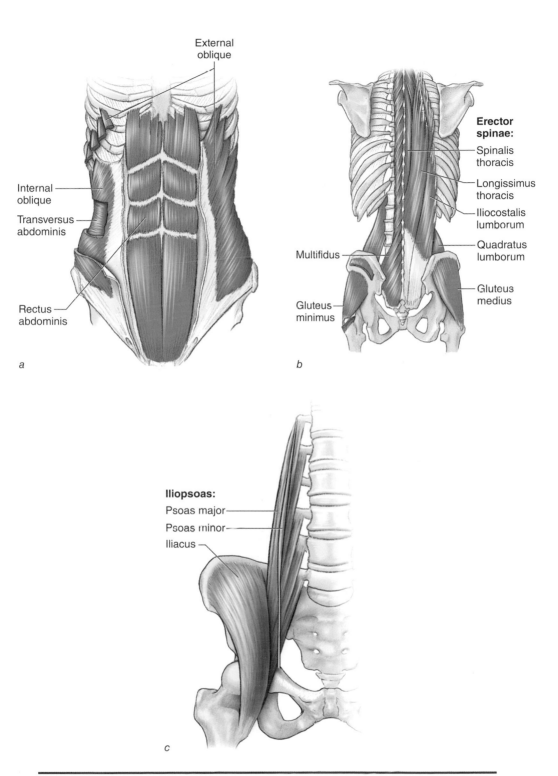

FIGURE 1.9 Core muscles: (a) abdominal muscles; (b) posterior outer core muscles; (c) anterior outer core muscles.

Three sheaths of muscles make up the core. The upper abdominal muscles move the body between the rib cage and the pelvis. In addition, the oblique abdominal muscles (obliques), which are positioned at the sides of the trunk, are essential for the twisting actions that mark many sports. Finally, a deep layer of abdominal muscles supports your internal organs. All three layers must be strong and work together to provide a balanced, effective yoga practice.

A strong core protects the low back and reduces injuries. The core also gives power to the legs for quick bursts of strength. In fact, core strength gives power, stability, and balance for greater performance in all sports, so it is important for everyone. A full yoga practice builds all the core muscles because the balance needed to hold the poses and stretches involves the deepest muscles of the body. Some yoga poses, such as the boat pose, focus directly on the core. This pose reminds you how important the core is in performance.

Boat Pose

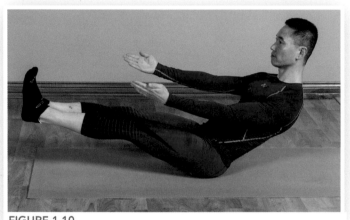

FIGURE 1.10

Muscles

Psoas, pectineus, sartorius, rectus femoris, rectus abdominis, adductors, quadriceps, erector spinae, quadratus lumborum, trapezius, rhomboids

1. Sit on your mat.
2. Bend your knees and plant your feet on the mat.
3. Wrap your hands around your thighs.
4. Lean your torso back until your arms are straight.
5. Lean back farther until your feet lift off the floor and you are balancing on your butt, just behind the sitting bones.

6. As you hold the pose, engage your core by pulling your navel toward your spine.
7. Straighten your legs (figure 1.10).
8. Keep lifting your chest to maintain a long spine and to keep your core engaged.
9. Gaze forward.

Modification

Enter the pose the same way, but keep your knees bent rather than extending the legs.

Safety Tip

Keep your chest lifted and your navel pulled in to strengthen your core and to avoid strain on your low back. Lifting the chest also helps to prevent a rounded back, which can contribute to pain and overuse injuries.

Improve Sleep

At times the mind races with thoughts that prevent you from relaxing and even getting to sleep. As a result, at some point in your life you may encounter insomnia. While sleepless nights can be troubling to everyone, they are particularly damaging to athletes who are preparing to perform; a good night's sleep is as essential as training. No perfect solution exists for occasional insomnia, but you can learn to relax. Relaxing is as much a skill as exerting your muscles, and yoga can help you train your body to relax. Yoga accomplishes this task in two ways. First, when you learn to concentrate on poses during your yoga practice, your mind and body learn to understand the difference between effort and relaxation. Later when you focus on relaxation, your muscles will be able to respond to the command to relax. This skill works on and off your mat; it can translate to your bed for restful sleep.

A second way yoga helps improve sleep is with breathing. Throughout your yoga practice you consciously use breath to help you get into and be in poses, and at the end of practice you use breath to calm down. To achieve a relaxing breath, start with deep breathing. Take slow, long, smooth inhalations and exhalations. On the inhalation, count 5 to 7 seconds, and count 5 to 10 seconds to exhale. Once you have established a rhythm with your breath, keep that flow for at least a minute, or as long as you feel completely relaxed and ready for sleep. Athletes use this rhythmic breathing before a game to calm down and relax so that they can perform at the highest level; it works before sleep as well. All yoga sessions end with relaxation pose (also called *savasana*, which is Sanskrit for "corpse pose"). Use this pose to practice the technique of relaxation so that you can transfer it to your daily life and improve your sleep.

Relaxation Pose

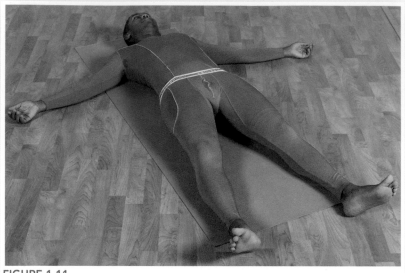

FIGURE 1.11

Muscles

No muscles are worked; you should be completely relaxed.

1. Lie on the mat on your back.
2. Extend your legs and relax them, letting your feet fall to the sides.
3. Lengthen your arms out to your sides with your palms facing up (figure 1.11).
4. Close your eyes.
5. Let go of any tension you are holding in your body.
6. Let your breath flow naturally.
7. Allow thoughts to pass through your mind, without holding on to them. As you let thoughts come and go, focus on relaxing.

Modifications

If any back discomfort occurs, bend both knees and plant your feet on your mat about hip-width apart or wider and relax your knees together. Another option as a great modification if being on your back is not comfortable is the seated cross-legged pose.

Yoga Safety

Yoga is not a competition. This concept is difficult to grasp particularly for competitive athletes, whose life is competition. However, when you are on your mat, you have to focus on your own body and what it can do rather than matching or beating what someone else might be able to do. You must even resist the urge to compete with yourself; it is best to stay focused on where you are today and not overstretch or overexert. Feel free to use props such as blocks and straps to help you safely achieve a pose. These tools are explained in chapter 2.

It is also important to stay hydrated before and during class, or you might feel light-headed or even dizzy. Keep water nearby so that you can take a drink. Yoga poses can be deceptively challenging, and even athletes need to be careful about their water intake. Just as in any athletic endeavor, maintaining proper form in the poses helps to prevent injuries, so read the instructions carefully and look at the pictures to make sure you are doing everything correctly.

Finally, if at any point in your practice you feel fatigued or light-headed, rest in child's pose for a moment. This pose is a restorative pose for the whole body and mind, and it allows you to check in with yourself during your yoga practice.

Child's Pose

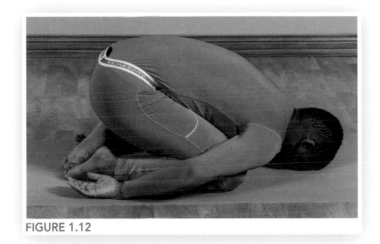

FIGURE 1.12

Muscles
Latissimus dorsi, erector spinae, gluteus maximus

1. Lower yourself to your hands and knees.
2. Bring your big toes together and knees apart.
3. Take your hips back to your heels.
4. Relax your forehead on the mat.
5. Lengthen your arms down along your sides, palms facing up (figure 1.12).

Modifications
Bring your knees together and extend your arms overhead. This will give your back a stretch and allow your shoulders to relax externally while extended overhead. If your knees hurt in this pose, come to seated cross-legged pose or put your legs up against the wall.

Safety Tip
You should not feel pain or discomfort in the knees. If you do, modify the pose as needed or practice seated cross-legged pose or legs up the wall pose.

Summary

Yoga is a wonderful complement for athletic training. Whether you are an amateur or professional athlete, a yoga practice will enhance your current athletic performance and help you have a long athletic career. The poses described in this chapter are only a sample to give you an idea of how yoga can improve your training. Now it is time to turn to a systematic practice. Chapters 2 and 3 start with basic and advanced warm-ups to begin your practice. Like all yoga practice, this is a journey—a journey to enhanced athletic performance.

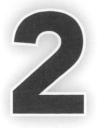

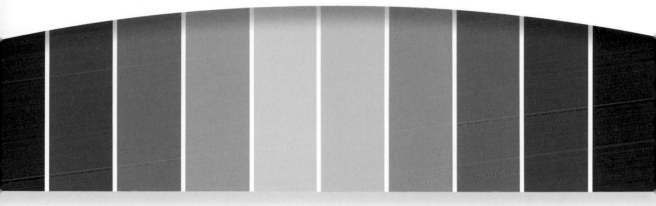

GETTING STARTED

Now that you know the benefits that yoga can bring to your sports performance, it's time to get started. Before you begin the poses in this chapter, aim to maintain correct form so that you can avoid injury. Athletes usually have well-developed muscles, so poses requiring flexibility may be challenging. To ease the challenge of getting into poses while maintaining proper form, try using the props shown in figure 2.1. Use these props to elevate the ground for support, to prevent you from slipping, as extension cords to reach your limbs, or to cushion parts of your body.

Here's what you might need:

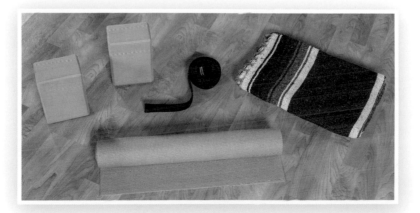

FIGURE 2.1   Yoga props.

Yoga Mat

Mats provide a surface that will let your hands and feet grip easily so that you won't slip as you are holding a pose. Mats come in different thicknesses. Some people like a thicker mat to give more padding, but padding can make balance poses more difficult. Other people like a thin mat so that they can feel the surface beneath. Experiment to see what you like. You can always stack two mats to get the surface that best suits you.

If your new mat is slippery, wash it in the bathtub with a small amount of detergent. Rinse it with vinegar and water to be sure the residue is gone. You can also wash it in a solution of baking soda and water. Some yoga mats are machine washable. If you wash yours in the machine, remove it before the spin cycle to avoid possible damage from stretching, then hang it to dry.

Always keep your mat clean. You should wipe it down between workouts to prevent any build-up of bacteria or oils from sweating. You can spray your mat with commercial yoga mat cleaners or make your own by filling a spray bottle with a little mild detergent, vinegar, and water. Wipe it down with a clean towel, and you are ready for your next workout. Some mat materials respond better to some cleaning products than others. Check the manufacturer's recommendations for maintaining your mat.

Two Yoga Blocks

At the beginning of a practice, your muscles may be too inflexible to let them reach the floor as you stretch for a pose. This inflexibility may cause you to do a pose incorrectly, creating misalignments in the body, which undercuts all the good the practice is doing. Blocks are useful tools for elevating the floor as your muscles slowly start to stretch.

Blocks are usually made of foam or cork. You can also find wood or bamboo blocks. The most common size is 3 inches (7.6 cm) long by 6 inches (15.2 cm) wide and 9 inches (22.8 cm) high. These measurements allow you to use various heights of a block depending on your level of flexibility. Foam blocks are the lightest and most commonly found in yoga studios.

If you don't have a block, use a stack of books, a piece of furniture, or anything else that can support the weight of your hand or your seat.

Yoga Strap

Like the blocks, straps can help us maintain proper form when stretching into a pose. Straps looped around our hands or feet will let us keep our spines long as we open our shoulders or hips while we are in folds or twists.

The most popular length for yoga straps is 6 feet (1.8 m), but tall people might want to use 8-foot (2.4-m) or even 10-foot (3-m) straps. The long straps are particularly useful for taller or larger athletes, such as basketball or football players.

Yoga straps come with fasteners at the end so that you can secure them as you hold a stretch. The two most popular kinds have either a plastic clip or a metal D-ring. Both work equally well; it is a matter of personal taste.

If you don't own a strap made for yoga, don't be afraid to improvise. You can use a twisted towel or a belt to help you achieve a pose.

Two-Inch Block, Bolster, or Blanket

If your hips are tight, sitting on the floor often curves the lower back, putting tension on the sacrum. Raising the sitting bones a bit relieves that strain and allows you bend forward to stretch the hamstrings without lower-back strain. The easiest way to accomplish this elevation is to sit on a two-inch (5-cm) block, bolster, or even a folded blanket or towel.

Throughout this book, you will see examples of athletes using these props in their practice. Feel free to use props in any poses as needed. You will soon come to know your own body so that you can decide for yourself when to use a prop. Remember, the goal is to achieve the proper form; it doesn't matter whether it is with a prop or not.

It All Starts With Your Breath

Breathing lies at the heart of athletic performance, and athletes instinctively know this fact whether they are conscious of it or not. Tennis players get the maximum power in their stroke if they exhale as they hit, and endurance swimmers and runners depend on rhythmic breathing to propel them along. This principle remains true for all sports. Trained athletes learn to use their breath without actively thinking about it.

PETER FLUCKE

Marathon Runner and Cyclist

I began practicing yoga years after my training and races to improve my flexibility and recovery from marathon and bicycle training. I was surprised to find the breathing and relaxation of yoga to be equally as valuable. Four marathons (including Boston) and two unsupported tandem bicycle rides across the country later, I can't imagine a life without yoga.

One of the key elements in yoga practice is becoming aware of our breathing and controlling the breath to enhance our performance. Yoga uses the Sanskrit term *pranayama* to refer to the practice of controlling the breath. The word means "extension of the breath," but it also means "extension of the life force," reinforcing the fact that the breath is at the heart of your life force. By consciously controlling breath during yoga practice, you will soon become aware of how much your breath influences your performance, and you can bring that knowledge and muscle–breath memory to your sport.

It is easy to hold your breath during periods of intense activity or deep stretches, because at these times you are concentrating on muscle effort. However, your true focus should be full, complete breaths that fuel your performance. Breathing supplies oxygen to the body, and oxygen nourishes cells and muscles. Blood flows to the muscles to supply nourishment and rid the muscle tissues of waste. This flow brings energy to the systems of the body to help regenerate and revitalize it. Breath builds stamina and endurance to improve athletic performance.

Yoga offers a number of breathing techniques to help enhance your yoga practice. A conscious breathing technique called ujjayi breath (*ujjayi* is Sanskrit for "victorious") is particularly good for athletes, and it is easy for all levels of yoga practitioners to learn.

To learn this technique, sit on the floor with your spine straight and your legs crossed. (If this position isn't comfortable because of tight hips, sit on a block or folded blanket to raise your hips above your knees so that you can straighten your spine.) Inhale through your nose, then open your mouth. As you exhale through your mouth, add a gentle whispering sound of *hhaaaa*. Feel a vibration of the air coming through your vocal chords. Do a few more rounds this way to practice the sound and breath. Once you can consistently feel the whispering of your breath, you are ready to move on.

To do the full ujjayi breathing, inhale through the nose and begin to exhale with an open mouth. Halfway through the exhalation, close your mouth, keeping the whispering *hhaaaa* sound. Continue with the flow of your breath and the whispering sound of ujjayi breath on both the inhalations and exhalations. With practice, this sound and flow of your breath will become more familiar and you will be using your ujjayi breath with no effort at all.

Now that you have the sound of the breathing, you can focus on attaining the proper form of the breath. The best deep breathing begins with your diaphragm, the strong muscle that lies at the bottom of your lungs. As you inhale, concentrate first on lowering your diaphragm as the air seems to fill your belly; it is really filling your lower lungs. Next, bring the air into your lower rib cage and finally to your upper chest. As you exhale, start again with your diaphragm, contracting it to force the air out of your lungs, out of your lower ribs, through the upper ribs and through the throat, leaving with the whisper of ujjayi breath as the air vibrates through your throat. Throughout your practice in the poses, concentrate on using this breathing technique. Soon it will become second nature. Your diaphragm will strengthen—it's a muscle, after all—and your breathing will enhance your athletic performance.

Warm-Up Exercises and Stretches

One of the most important benefits yoga can bring to athletes is flexibility to keep their muscles supple. Most people don't hold their stretches long enough to do any good. Holding stretches lengthens the muscles, which increases muscle flexibility and joint range of motion. You should hold your stretch for 20 seconds to a full minute, and even longer if your muscles are tight and you can relax into the stretch. It may seem like a long time, but if you focus on your ujjayi breathing instead of the muscle tension, the exercise will be more effective. Some athletes like to count their breaths to be sure they hold long enough.

Do not bounce while stretching. Bouncing doesn't improve flexibility, and it can lead to tiny tears in muscle tissue. If these tears occur, muscles can create scar tissue as they heal. Scar tissue can lead to more pain and less flexibility in the muscles, undoing any good you might have done. So, simply hold that stretch and breathe deeply.

Following are some basic yoga moves to get you started. These warm-ups will wake up your body, letting it know it is time to start working out safely before you move on to a more vigorous practice.

Half Happy Baby Pose

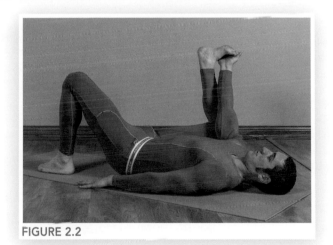

FIGURE 2.2

Muscles

Gluteus maximus and hamstrings on the bent leg; flexors, psoas, sartorius, adductor longus and brevis, rectus femoris, and pectineus on the straight leg

1. Lie on your back.
2. Pull one knee to your chest, and keeping the knee bent, place the opposite foot on the mat.
3. Reach your arm to the inside of your bent leg (figure 2.2).

(continued)

4. Reach over the top of your ankle, and clasp the outer edge of your foot.
5. Lift your foot up toward the ceiling.
6. Press down on your right foot, working your right knee toward the floor. Keep pressing down from the foot, working the knee toward the floor next to your shoulder.
7. Lengthen the straight leg long through the heel while pressing the hamstring down toward the floor as you keep the foot flexed.
8. Hold the posture for 5 to 10 breaths.
9. Repeat the pose on the other side.

Modification

If your hips and hip flexors are really tight, wrap a strap around the ball of the right foot and pull down on the strap, taking the knee toward the floor next to your right shoulder. Bend your left knee and plant the left foot on the mat. This action will provide space to get into this pose.

Safety Tip

If you have knee problems from past injuries, make sure you do not feel any pain or discomfort in your knees. If you do, hug your right knee into your chest without adding pressure to the foot, and lengthen your left leg down to your mat.

Supine Spinal Twist

Muscles

Gluteus maximus, gluteus medius, tensor fasciae latae, hamstrings, pectoralis major, biceps, brachialis

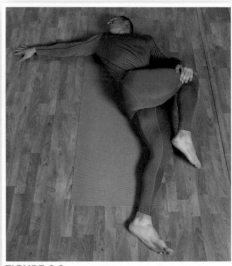

FIGURE 2.3

1. Warming up the back is important, especially if you are naturally tight or a little achy in the back. Spinal twists are a great way to wake up the back muscles and improve the flexibility of the spine.
2. Lie on your back.
3. Pull your right knee to your chest.
4. Extend your right arm to your side and down to the floor.
5. With your left hand, guide your right knee to the left toward the floor and lift your right hip off the ground.
6. Look to your right as you hold this pose. Reach your right arm to the right, keeping at least your right palm or back of your hand touching the floor (figure 2.3).

7. Hold the posture for 5 breaths.
8. Repeat the twist with the left leg, looking to your left.

Modification

Keep your knee to your chest and only lower the knee part way as comfortable, squeezing it in tightly (figure 2.4).

Safety Tip

Avoid this pose if you experience back pain. Instead, hug one knee into your chest and repeat the posture on the other side.

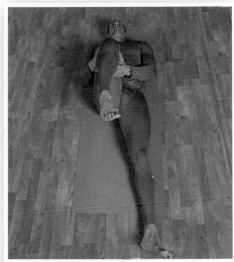

FIGURE 2.4 Supine spinal twist modification.

Cat/Cow

Muscles

Abdominal muscles, erector spinae, quadratus lumborum, trapezius

1. Start on your hands and knees with your hands under your shoulders and knees under your hips.
2. Inhale as you drop your belly and lift your chin and tailbone up toward the sky (figure 2.5a).
3. As you exhale, tuck your chin to your chest, tuck your tailbone under, press into your palms to keep your arms straight, and arch your upper back toward the sky (figure 2.5b).
4. Move with your breath. This movement is not only good for your back, it also warms up your neck and hips. This movement of the spine is good for forward folding poses and an easy backbend to help continue with your warm-up.

Safety Tip

If you feel any discomfort in the back, try moving more slowly. While moving in this pose, keep the belly slightly engaged on the inhalation to prevent strain on the back.

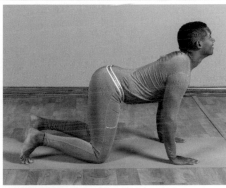

FIGURE 2.5a

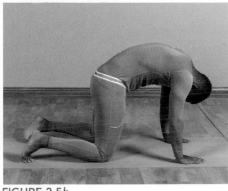

FIGURE 2.5b

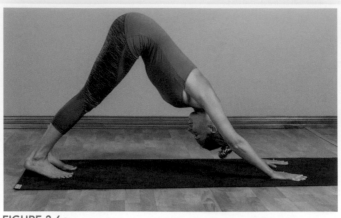

FIGURE 2.6a

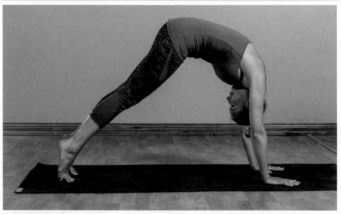

FIGURE 2.6b

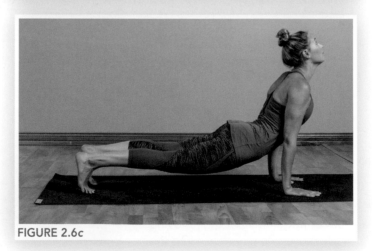

FIGURE 2.6c

Muscles

Triceps, hamstrings, gastrocnemius, soleus, quadratus lumborum, erector spinae, trapezius, abdominal muscles, pectoralis

1. Spine rolling pulls together the warm-up through a fluid movement with the breath to help warm up the whole body.
2. Start in downward-facing dog pose (see chapter 1; figure 2.6*a*).
3. Lift your heels high, and tuck your chin to your chest (figure 2.6*b*).
4. Exhale completely.
5. Inhaling, tuck your tailbone under. Round your spine forward and through to upward-facing dog pose (see chapter 1; figure 2.6*c*), and lift your chin slightly.
6. As you exhale, tuck your chin to your chest and round your spine as you move back to downward-facing dog pose.
7. Alternate between poses by moving with the breath for 3 to 6 rounds.

Modifications

From downward-facing dog pose, shift forward to a high push-up position (plank pose). Lower your hips toward the floor, pressing your hands into the floor, lengthening your arms and lifting your chest to upward-facing dog pose. Another option is to stay in downward-facing dog pose, pressing your heels down into the mat or toward the mat.

Safety Tip

If you have any discomfort in the shoulders or low back, it is best to do the modified version. This movement requires strength in the upper body, so be aware of how the back and shoulders move and feel.

Summary

You now have some foundational knowledge of yoga. You know which props to use, how to breathe, and how to do some preliminary warm-up poses. These simple stretches have warmed up your muscles, alerting them that you are ready to work out. The following chapters focus on poses specifically for the athletic body. You are strong and motivated to improve your performance, so it is time to move on. Always remember to focus on your breathing and look carefully at the safety tips that are included. Now it's time for full-body warm-ups.

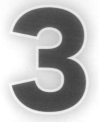

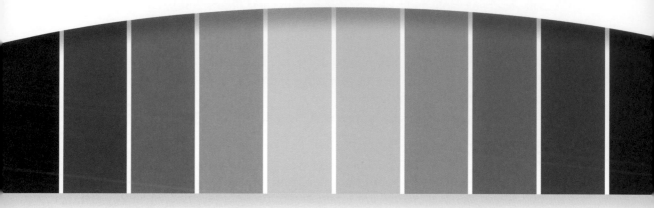

WARMING UP

Chapter 2 introduced gentle poses to awaken the joints and prepare muscles for movement. This chapter describes sun salutations (called *surya namaskara* in Sanskrit), a series of full-body poses that will prepare athletes for the specific stretches needed to improve performance. Sun salutations stretch and strengthen all the muscles and stimulate blood flow throughout the body, so it is always worthwhile to begin a practice with this series of poses.

Beginning yoga practitioners often find these sequences challenging because they require a measure of upper-body strength. However, athletes tend to be strong, so they can flow through these sequences once they learn the moves. For athletes, the concern is not so much strength building through yoga but gaining flexibility and balance. These full-body sequences not only warm up the muscles, they develop balance and start the process of stretching for flexibility. Flowing between poses reinforces the idea that the nature of sports is movement.

Before you begin the sequences, remember your ujjayi breathing. Use deep breaths from the diaphragm to the ribs to the upper chest, and listen to the oceanlike whispering sound of your breath as you flow

MIKE NEAL
NFL Linebacker

Visualization has been very effective for me. Being a professional athlete, you have to be able to visualize things before they happen, to watch plays be made beforehand. Visualization helps create a positive imagery environment. To me, this visualization is a substantial part of a successful career. The more positive visualization you put into the universe, the more positivity you get back! Visualization and faith go hand in hand for me. They have the same underlying theme of believing in things before you actually see them come to pass. Yoga has helped me create a positive environment. It has also taught me to use visualization. Being able to breathe deeply and release the tension of the world though yoga helped me obtain peace and create a positive environment for my mind. It was once said, "You change your thoughts, you change your life." I recommend trying visualization as often as possible!

through the movements. Be sure to fill your lungs completely to get the full effect of ujjayi breathing. You are working your lungs and diaphragm throughout this sequence. The sequence of breathing is described for each pose—inhale through one pose, and exhale through one pose—but after you go through the sequence once or twice, you should be able to follow the breath automatically. Remember, the discipline of your breath will enhance the flow of your body.

Athletic Variation

In many flow series, you will step back (e.g., into a plank pose) or step forward (e.g., when moving from plank pose to a forward fold). To build arm strength or use arm strength to develop balance (as many athletes do), instead of stepping back into plank or stepping forward to bring the feet between the hands, you can jump to the position. Jumping back and forward requires you to lift your hips, bringing your weight over your hands. When jumping with the weight in the hands, keep your shoulders firm.

Figure 3.1 shows the proper alignment of the hips over the shoulders to minimize risk of shoulder injury. Note that you have to tighten your core as you exhale and lift your hips to achieve this position.

Jumping Hips Up

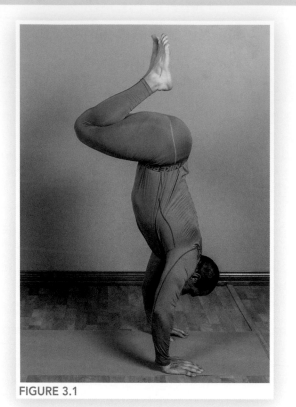
FIGURE 3.1

Muscles

Biceps, deltoids, trapezius, pectoralis major and minor

1. Start in downward-facing dog pose.
2. Walk your feet next to each other.
3. Take one step forward with both feet so that your feet are a step closer to your hands.
4. Deeply bend your knees.
5. Look between your hands.
6. Exhale completely.
7. Push from your feet to lift your hips high above your shoulders as you jump forward (figure 3.1).
8. Grip the mat with your fingertips.
9. Broaden your shoulders.
10. Slowly lower your feet between your hands.

Modification

Instead of jumping, simply step both feet between your hands.

Safety Tip

Follow the modification if jumping is not in your practice.

Sun Salutation A

The sun salutations are sequences that flow together with the breath, using a number of muscles throughout the body to help build heat in the body for your practice. It is always good to do four to six rounds of sun salutations to fully warm up your body. Sun salutations have several variations, but athletes should begin with sun salutation A.

Muscles

Serratus anterior, rhomboids, pectoralis major, pectoralis minor, deltoids, triceps, infraspinatus, teres minor, rectus abdominis, transverse abdominis, gluteus maximus, gluteus minimus, erector spinae, trapezius, hamstrings (semitendinosus, semimembranosus, biceps femoris), calves, (gastrocnemius, soleus), psoas, quadriceps (rectus femoris, vastus lateralis, vastus intermedius, vastus medialis), quadratus lumborum

1 Begin in mountain pose (figure 3.2). Stand at the top of your mat with your big toes touching and heels slightly apart. Your body weight should be evenly distributed on the bottoms of your feet. Keep your knees slightly unlocked to avoid hyperextension. Stack your hips above your knees and ankles. Drop your tailbone between your heels, and draw your rib cage slightly in and downward. Pull your shoulders back and your shoulder blades down your back. Stand tall with your arms down along your sides and your palms facing forward. Feel tall through the top of your head; imagine a string pulling you to the ceiling. Hold this position for 3 breaths. **Modification:** If it's not comfortable to have the big toes touch, place your feet about hip-width apart or closer. If you feel rounded forward, stand with your heels next to a wall and lean into the wall. Press your shoulders back into the wall and the shoulder blades down your back. Tuck your tailbone toward your heels as you slightly pull your rib cage in toward the midline of the body. Place the back of your head into the wall as you extend your arms down, and gently press the backs of your hands into the wall. Lengthen tall through the top of your head. **Safety tip:** Avoid hyperextension in the knees.

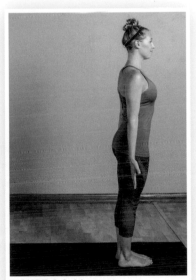

FIGURE 3.2 Mountain pose.

(continued)

2 From mountain pose, move into mountain pose with arms overhead (figure 3.3). Start in mountain pose. Inhale as you raise both arms overhead until your palms touch. Maintain your mountain pose with the arms overhead. Take 1 breath. **Modification:** Keep your arms down along your sides. **Safety tip:** Avoid hyperextension in the knees.

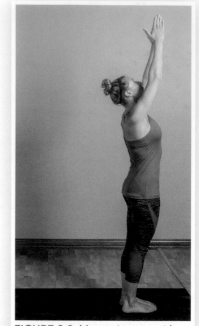

FIGURE 3.3 Mountain pose with arms overhead.

3 From mountain pose with arms overhead, move into forward fold (figure 3.4). As you exhale, lengthen your arms and chest forward as you hinge at the hips. Do not round your back. Fold toward the floor, letting your chest fall toward your thighs while keeping your legs straight and relaxing your neck. Place your hands next to your feet. Hold the posture for 1 breath. **Modification:** Before forward folding, bend at the knees. Move into the forward fold and wrap your arms around your legs, hugging your legs into your chest. Work on straightening your legs and lifting your hips toward the sky for a deeper hamstring stretch. **Safety tip:** You do not want to strain the back when reaching the arms forward. To prevent back strain, place your hands on your thighs and keep a deep bend in both knees to slowly fold forward. Wrap both arms around the legs.

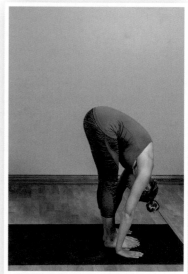

FIGURE 3.4 Forward fold.

4 From forward fold, move into a flat back (figure 3.5). Inhale as you lift your torso to a flat back (halfway up to standing). Keeping your legs straight, place your fingertips in front of the toes and lengthen the spine and chest forward. Slide your shoulder blades down your back. Push your shoulders down away from your ears to allow the collarbones to broaden and the spine to lengthen forward. Hold the posture for 1 breath. ***Modification:*** If your hamstrings restrict you from keeping a flat back, place your hands on your shins or on a couple of blocks. This modification will help maintain a flat back as you lengthen your spine forward. Your gaze should be straight ahead. If you still feel a strain on the hamstrings with the hands on the shins or blocks, slightly bend both knees while maintaining a flat back. ***Safety tip:*** Maintain bent knees to prevent any back pain.

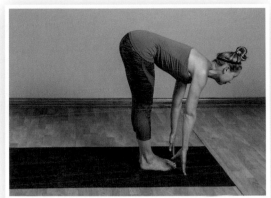

FIGURE 3.5 Flat back.

5 From flat back, move into plank pose (figure 3.6). Plant your palms on the mat and step both feet back to a high push-up position. Tighten your core and buttocks to stay strong in your center. Separate your fingers, and press your palms down into the mat. Keep your arms straight and shoulders down away from your ears. Keep your whole body long by lengthening back through your heels and forward through the top of your head. Take 1 breath. ***Modification:*** This pose takes strength in the upper body and core, so if it is too difficult to maintain, lower both knees to the floor while maintaining a long spine and keeping your shoulders away from your ears. ***Safety tip:*** Avoid creating any discomfort in your shoulders and wrists. If you do feel any pain, practice the cat/cow movement described in chapter 2 instead of plank pose.

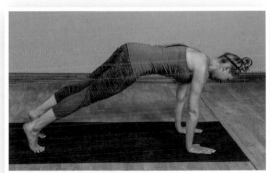

FIGURE 3.6 Plank pose.

(continued)

6 From plank pose, move into four-limbed staff pose (known in Sanskrit as *cha-turanga dandasana*; figure 3.7). Beginners usually dislike this pose, and athletes usually love it, both for the same reason; it is a strength pose! To get into four-limbed staff pose, begin in plank pose. Exhaling, slowly lower halfway to the floor as you tip slightly forward to align your shoulders, elbows, and wrists at a 90-degree angle (figure 3.7). Keep your elbows tight to your sides by pulling your shoulder blades down your back. Engage your core to help maintain a long body without dipping your chest or hips. Slightly push your heels back, and at the same time pull your collarbones forward to lengthen the whole body. Take 1 breath. ***Modification:*** Lower your knees to the floor, then follow the other instructions for chaturanga dandasana. ***Safety tip:*** Keep the body in line. Do not lower the head or hips first. Keeping the body lined up will allow you to use your muscles and keep you away from injuring your shoulders, wrists, and back.

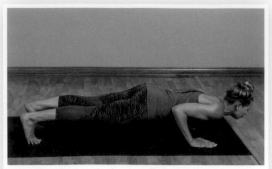

FIGURE 3.7 Four-limbed staff pose.

7 From four-limbed staff pose, move into upward-facing dog pose (figure 3.8). Inhale as you lift your chest and straighten your arms. Roll over your toes to the tops of your feet. Press the tops of your feet down into your mat as you engage your quadriceps and lift your knees off the floor, maintaining a slight engagement of your gluteal muscles. Keep your shoulders down and back, moving away from your ears. Keep your palms pressing down into your mat to maintain straight arms. Gaze forward to relax your neck. Pull your shoulder blades down your back; your shoulders push back as your shoulder blades press down. The shoulders and wrists should be lined up. Take 1 breath. ***Modification:*** If this pose is too intense for your shoulders, wrists, or spine, perform cobra pose. Lower to your belly. Place your palms on the mat under your shoulders. Keep your elbows bent and pointed up toward the sky.

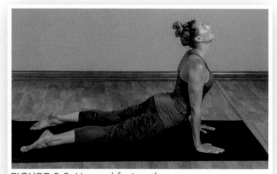

FIGURE 3.8 Upward-facing dog pose.

Gently press your palms into the mat just enough to pull your chest forward and up, lifting halfway up. The tops of your feet stay on the mat. Tuck your tailbone toward your feet to keep your back long and avoid sinking into your low back. **Safety tip:** Keep your core slightly engaged to prevent discomfort in your low back. If you have low-back or any shoulder problems, it would be best to do cobra pose instead of upward-facing dog pose.

8 From upward-facing dog pose, move into downward-facing dog pose (figure 3.9). Exhale as you lift your hips up and back, rolling over your toes. Press into your hands to lengthen your arms. Make sure your hands are shoulder-width apart and your pointer fingers point to the top of your mat. Separate the fingers so that they spread wide. Externally roll your shoulders out and away from your ears. It is easy to shrug your shoulders in this pose, so counter that action by pulling the shoulders toward the middle of the back. Relax your neck. Firmly and evenly across your palms, press into your mat to help lengthen your spine and lift your hips. Lengthen your legs as you straighten your legs and press your heels down into or toward the mat. Hold the pose for 5 breaths. **Modification:** If your hamstrings are tight and your spine rounds, bend both knees slightly. Focus on a long spine by pressing into your palms and lifting your hips. **Safety tip:** Watch for any hyperextension. In this pose, it is easy to hyperextend the elbows and knees.

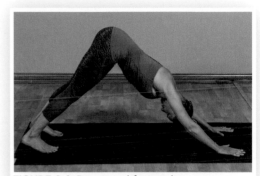
FIGURE 3.9 Downward-facing dog pose.

9 From downward-facing dog pose, move again into a flat back (figure 3.10). Inhale as you step the feet forward between the hands. Place your big toes together, heels slightly apart. Place your fingers on the floor in front of your feet. Lift your chest halfway up, and lengthen your spine forward to a flat back. Hold the position for 1 breath.

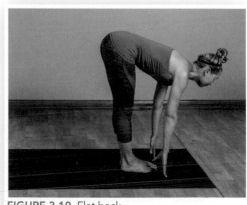
FIGURE 3.10 Flat back.

(continued)

10 From a flat back, move again into forward fold (figure 3.11). Exhale as you fold from your hips, taking your chest toward your thighs as you keep your legs straight. Place your hands on the floor next to your feet. Hold the pose for 1 breath.

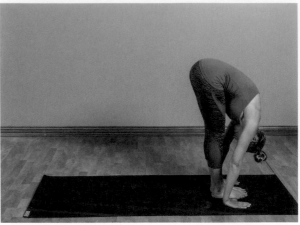

FIGURE 3.11 Forward fold.

11 From forward fold, rise into mountain pose with arms overhead (figure 3.12). Inhaling, extend your arms out as you lift your chest up. Come to standing as your palms touch overhead. Take 1 breath.

12 From mountain pose with arms overhead, finish in mountain pose (figure 3.13). Stand at the top of your mat with your feet together, arms overhead. Exhale fully as you lower your arms down along your sides. Take 1 breath.

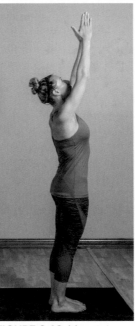

FIGURE 3.12 Mountain pose with arms overhead.

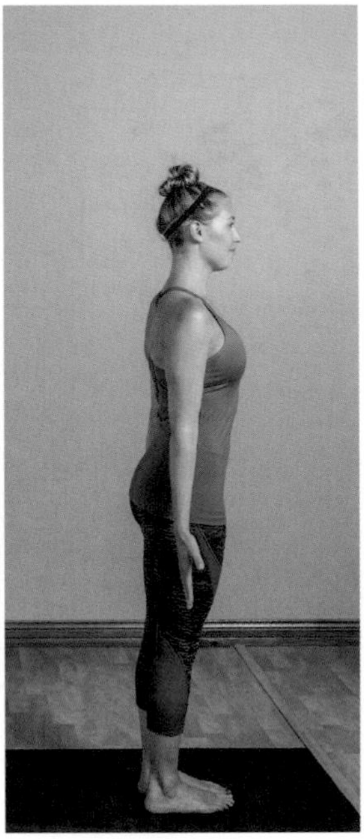

FIGURE 3.13 Mountain pose.

Sun Salutation B

Once you have repeated sun salutation A several times, you can move on to sun salutation B while flowing with the breath the same way as you did in Sun Salutation A. It is a similar sequence with a closed-leg squat to use the gluteal muscles, core, and quadriceps muscles on the fronts of the legs. The athletic variation applies here, too; you can step or jump back to plank just as you did in sun salutation A.

Sun salutations move through a cycle. You repeat the positions, returning to mountain pose in reverse order from the way you moved through to downward-facing dog pose. The sequence includes a rise and fall of the body and the breath, and this flow is what gives the body its full warm-up. Move rhythmically, and breathe deeply and regularly to get the maximum benefit of these poses. Many people consider these sequences to be a full workout, but for most athletes they serve as full-body warm-ups.

Muscles

Quadriceps (vastus medialis, vastus lateralis, rectus femoris, vastus intermedius), adductors, gluteus maximus, deltoids, pectoralis minor, serratus anterior, rectus abdominis, triceps, infraspinatus, teres minor, rhomboids, trapezius, erector spinae, quadratus lumborum, hamstrings (semitendinosus, semimembranosus, biceps femoris), calves (gastrocnemius, soleus), hip flexors, psoas, tibialis anterior, gluteus minimus, pectoralis major

1 Begin in mountain pose with the legs together. Stand tall, as shown in figure 3.14.

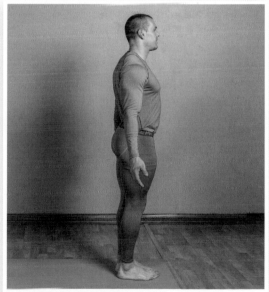

FIGURE 3.14 Mountain pose.

(continued)

2 From mountain pose, move into chair pose (figure 3.15). Inhaling, bend your knees, sinking your hips back and down as if you were sitting in a chair. Feel your weight on your heels as you relax your toes. Raise your arms, keeping your arms shoulder-width apart and slightly forward from your ears. Notice how your knees are together and you are working the quadriceps. Lift your chest, and relax your shoulders down so that you don't round your back. Keep your hips back and your tailbone tucked toward your heels while the chest lifts, maintaining a long spine to stay out of your lower back. Take 1 breath. **Modification:** Hold your palms together in prayer pose, thumbs touching your breastbone. Focus on the squat for this pose. **Safety tip:** Tight shoulders can cause strain on the neck, so relax the arms in prayer pose. Place a yoga block between your thighs to activate the inner thighs.

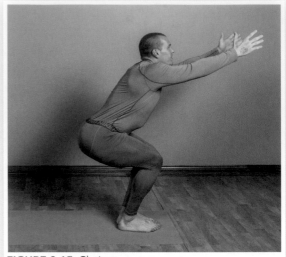

FIGURE 3.15 Chair pose.

3 From chair pose, move into forward fold (figure 3.16). Exhale as you fold your torso, taking your chest to your thighs straightening your legs.

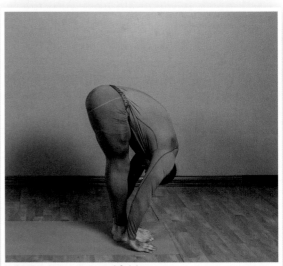

FIGURE 3.16 Forward fold.

4 From forward fold, move into a flat back (figure 3.17). Inhale while lifting your torso halfway up. Keep your hands on the floor or on your shins.

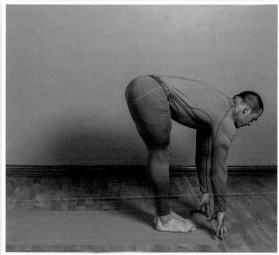

FIGURE 3.17 Flat back.

5 From flat back, move into plank pose (figure 3.18). Holding the inhalation, step or jump your feet back to plank pose.

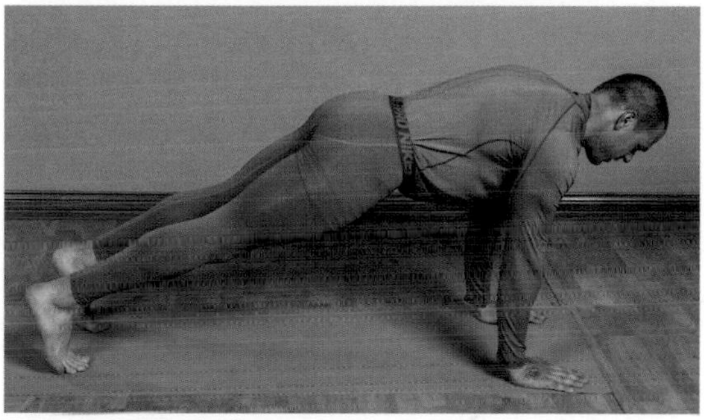

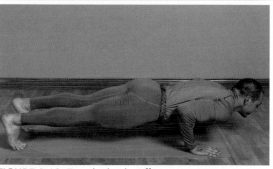

FIGURE 3.18 Plank pose.

6 From plank pose, move into four-limbed staff pose (figure 3.19). Exhaling, lower yourself halfway or all the way to the floor. Be sure to keep your elbows tight into your sides and use your back and abdominal muscles to lower yourself so that you reduce the risk of shoulder injury. Drop your knees if you need to modify the transition.

FIGURE 3.19 Four-limbed staff pose.

(continued)

7 From four-limbed staff pose, move into upward-facing dog pose (figure 3.20). As you inhale, roll forward to the tops of your feet. As you press your hands and feet down, lift your chest. Engage your thighs to lift them off the floor so to avoid putting any pressure on your lower back. **Modification:** Instead of upward-facing dog pose, move into cobra pose. Lower to your belly. Place your palms on the mat under your shoulders. Keep your elbows bent and pointed up toward the sky. Gently press your palms into the mat just enough to pull your chest forward and upward, lifting halfway up. Keep the tops of your feet on the mat. Tuck your tailbone toward your feet to keep your back long and avoid sinking into your low back.

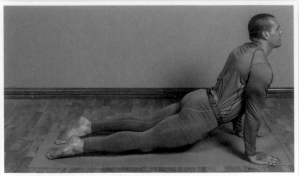

FIGURE 3.20 Upward-facing dog pose.

8 From upward-facing dog pose, move into downward-facing dog pose (figure 3.21). Exhaling, roll over your toes to lift your hips up and back. Press down into your palms to lengthen your spine up and back. Now, let's add a variation that did not exist with sun salutation A.

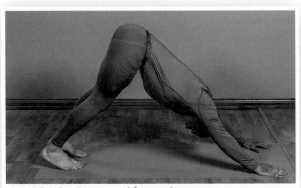

FIGURE 3.21 Downward-facing dog pose.

9 From downward-facing dog pose, move into three-legged downward-facing dog pose (figure 3.22). As you inhale, sweep your right leg up toward the sky. Lift your leg straight up through the heel, keeping your hips squared or opening the right hip a little. Keep your palms flat on the floor, and straighten the arms. Try to keep your shoulders squared to the front of your mat. For some people, keeping the hips square may be more difficult because of tight hip flexors, quadriceps, and hips. Lifting the leg up and opening your hip slightly will allow the space to lift

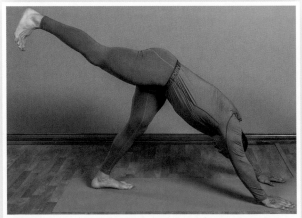

FIGURE 3.22 Three-legged downward-facing dog pose, right leg.

the leg and offer an added stretch. Take 1 breath with the right leg in the air; you will add the left leg later in the sequence. **Modification:** Lift your leg part of the way up if your hips and quadriceps are tight and restricting you. **Safety tip:** You should not feel any tension in the back. If you do, it is best to not lift your leg up to the ceiling. Just inhale as you remain in your downward-facing dog pose.

10 From three-legged downward-facing dog pose, move into warrior I pose on the right side (figure 3.23). Exhale as you step your right foot forward behind your right hand and place your left heel down. Bend your right knee, keeping it aligned above your right ankle. The hips remain facing forward throughout this pose. Imagine your hip bones as headlights facing forward. Make sure your feet are separated about hip width; don't line them up as if you were standing on a tightrope. Inhale as you lengthen your arms up just in front of your ears and lift your torso, looking forward. Hold for 1 breath. **Modification:** Keep your hands in prayer pose if raising your arms irritates the shoulders. If you experience any knee discomfort, straighten the front leg. **Safety tip:** Keep the core slightly engaged to maintain a long spine. You should not feel any shoulder or knee discomfort.

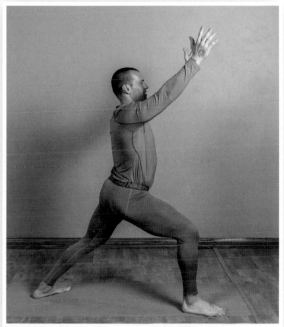

FIGURE 3.23 Warrior I pose, right side.

11 From warrior I, move into plank pose by releasing your hands to the floor. Step back to plank pose (figure 3.24).

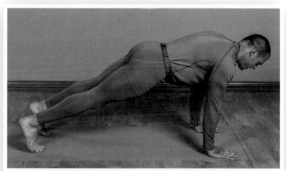

FIGURE 3.24 Plank pose.

12 From plank pose, move into four-limbed staff pose (figure 3.25). Lower yourself halfway (or all the way for the modified version) as you fully exhale.

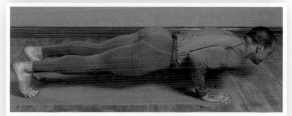

FIGURE 3.25 Four-limbed staff pose.

13 From four-limbed staff pose, move into upward-facing dog pose (figure 3.26). Inhale as you roll over your toes, press into your hands and feet, and lift up your chest. Engage your thighs to lift them off the floor. **Modification:** Instead of upward-facing dog pose, move into cobra pose.

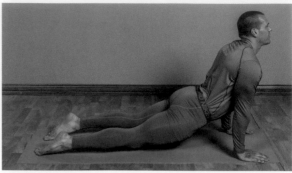

FIGURE 3.26 Upward-facing dog pose.

14 From upward-facing dog pose or cobra pose, move into downward-facing dog pose (figure 3.27). Exhale as you roll over your toes and lift your hips up and back. Hold the pose for 5 deep breaths.

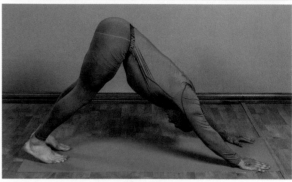

FIGURE 3.27 Downward-facing dog pose.

15 From downward-facing dog pose, move into three-legged downward-facing dog pose, lifting the left leg (figure 3.28 shows the right leg in the air for reference only). As you inhale, lift the left leg and repeat the series from three-legged downward facing dog. This time, your left leg goes up to the sky with the correct hip placement.

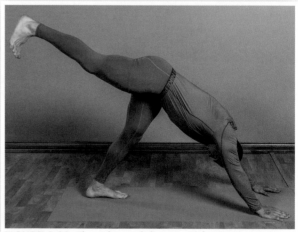

FIGURE 3.28 Three-legged downward-facing dog pose.

16 From three-legged downward-facing dog pose, move into warrior I pose on the left side (figure 3.29). Exhaling, bring your left leg behind your left hand and lower your left heel, then lift your torso and your arms as you did on the right side.

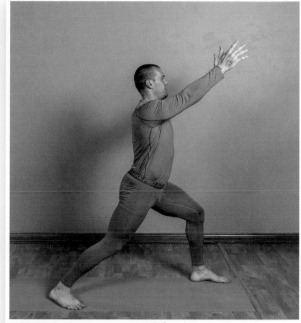

FIGURE 3.29 Warrior I pose, left side.

17 From warrior I pose on the left side, move into plank pose (figure 3.30). As you exhale, release your hands down to the floor and step your feet back.

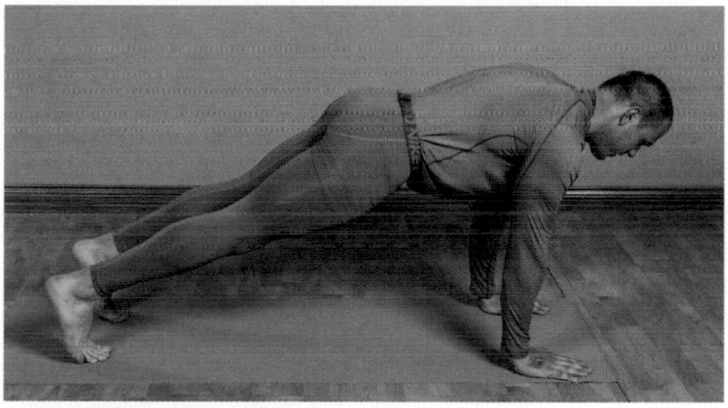

FIGURE 3.30 Plank pose.

18 From plank pose, move into four-limbed staff pose (figure 3.31). Exhaling, lower your body either halfway or all the way to the floor.

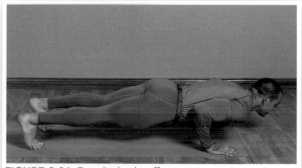

FIGURE 3.31 Four-limbed staff pose.

(continued)

19 From four-limbed staff pose, move into upward-facing dog pose (figure 3.32). Inhale as you roll over your toes. Press your hands and feet into the floor, lifting your chest. ***Modification:*** Move into cobra pose instead of upward-facing dog pose.

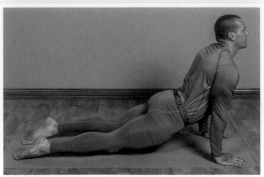

FIGURE 3.32 Upward-facing dog pose.

20 From upward-facing dog pose, move into downward-facing dog pose (figure 3.33). As you exhale, lift your hips up and back. Roll over your feet and lengthen your spine, lowering your heels toward the ground.

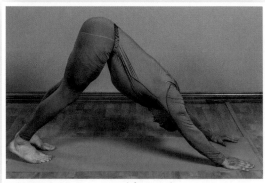

FIGURE 3.33 Downward-facing dog pose.

21 From downward-facing dog pose, move into hips over shoulders (3.34). Exhale completely as you look forward, then step or jump your hips over your shoulders, landing the feet between your hands.

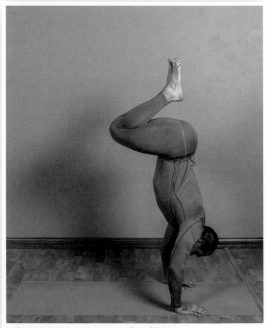

FIGURE 3.34 Hips over shoulders.

22 From hips over shoulders, move into a flat back (figure 3.35). Inhale while lifting your torso halfway up with your fingertips on the floor in front of your feet.

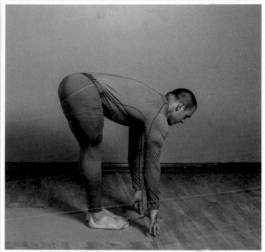
FIGURE 3.35 Flat back.

23 From flat back, move into forward fold (figure 3.36). Exhale as you take your chest to your thighs and straighten your legs, lowering your hands to the ground.

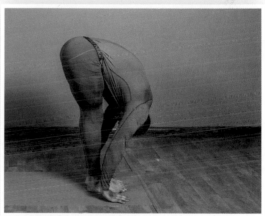
FIGURE 3.36 Forward fold.

24 From forward fold, move into chair pose (figure 3.37). Inhale as you bend your knees and sit your hips back. Raise your arms, keeping your arms shoulder-width apart and slightly forward from your ears.

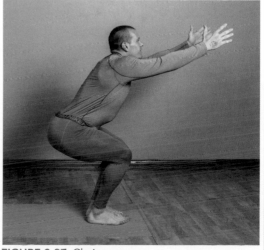
FIGURE 3.37 Chair pose.

25 From chair pose, finish in mountain pose (figure 3.38). Exhaling, straighten your legs and stand tall with your arms at your sides.

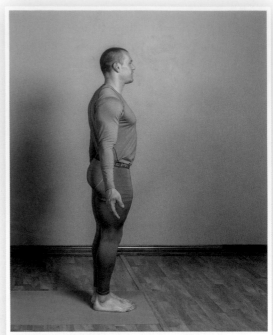

FIGURE 3.38 Mountain pose.

Variations for Sun Salutations

All exercises, including yoga poses, must be kept fresh and interesting. This rule applies especially to athletes, who are used to challenging their bodies. If you have the strength and energy for extra variations in your sun salutations, use the following variations to enhance your yoga practice and help build more heat in your body.

Double Four-Limbed Staff Pose

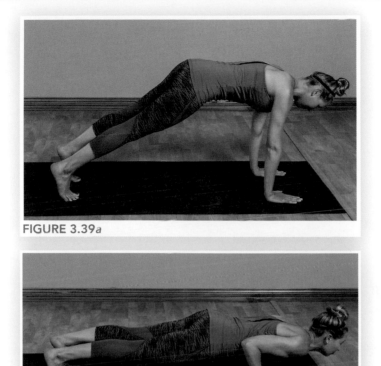

FIGURE 3.39*a*

FIGURE 3.39*b*

Muscles

Pectoralis major, pectoralis minor, serratus anterior, triceps, rectus abdominis, psoas, gluteus maximus, deltoids

1. Begin in plank pose (figure 3.39*a*). Keep your whole body long by lengthening forward through your collarbones and pushing back through your heels.
2. Squeeze your core by lifting your navel up toward your spine.
3. Squeeze your gluteal muscles.
4. Keep your shoulders back and away from your ears.
5. Exhale as you lower yourself down halfway (figure 3.39*b*).
6. Maintain the full-body engagement.
7. Inhaling, slowly push yourself back up, keeping your body straight.
8. Maintain the length and engagement of your body.
9. Do this sequence two times before you move into upward-facing dog pose.

Modification

Lower your knees to the ground.

Safety Tip

Don't do this sequence if you have shoulder and low-back issues. Instead, hold plank pose variation with your arms straight and knees on the floor.

Side Plank Pose

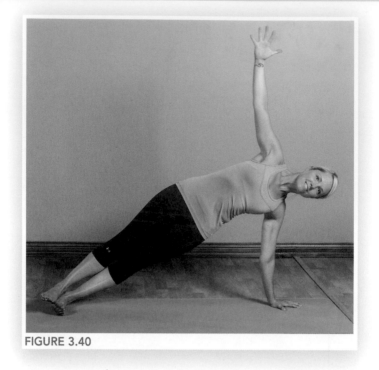

FIGURE 3.40

Muscles

Transversus abdominis, obliques, deltoid, gluteus medius, gluteus minimus, adductors (pectineus, adductor brevis, adductor longus, gracilis, adductor magnus)

1. While holding plank pose, put your weight onto your left hand.
2. Turn your body to balance on the outer edge of your left foot.
3. Stack your right foot on top of your left foot, and roll your right hip and shoulder back to stack up with your left hip and shoulder.
4. Reach your right arm to the ceiling (figure 3.40).
5. Press your shoulders down your back so that you don't put pressure on your neck.
6. Keep your body in line.
7. To transition to the right side, plant your right palm on the floor.
8. Roll to the outer edge of your right foot.
9. Stack your feet, hips, and shoulders.
10. Lengthen the left arm up to the ceiling.
11. Inhale, then as you exhale continue into four-limbed staff pose and through the rest of the sun salutation.

Modifications

Lower your forearm to the floor, and do a side plank pose on your forearm. Or lower your knee to the floor and do a side plank with your hand and knee to the floor.

Safety Tip

You should not feel any pain in your shoulders while doing this pose. If you do, follow the modification.

Three-Legged Downward-Facing Dog Pose With Core Work

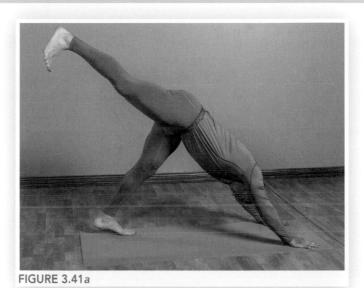

FIGURE 3.41a

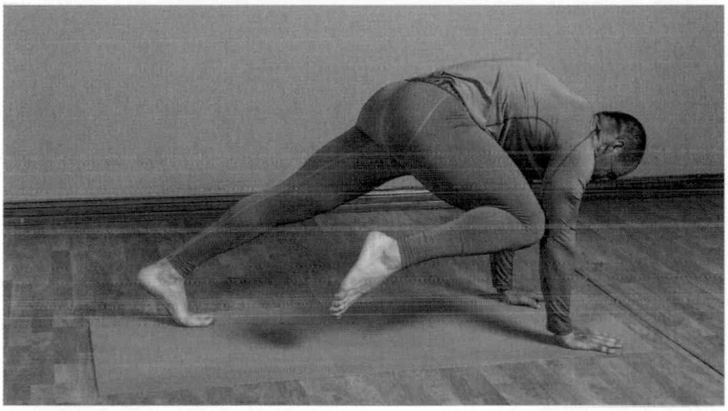

FIGURE 3.41b

Muscles

Triceps brachii, anterior deltoid, serratus anterior, latissimus dorsi, gluteus maximus, hamstrings (semitendinosus, biceps femoris, semimembranosus), iliopsoas, pectineus, tensor fasciae latae, vastus lateralis, pectoralis major, rectus abdominis, transverse abdominis, internal and external obliques

1. When you are in downward-facing dog pose in the middle of your sun salutation, add this sequence to increase your core strength. From downward-facing dog pose, inhale as you lift your right leg to the ceiling (figure 3.41a).

2. Exhaling, shift forward to plank pose as you bend your right knee to your right triceps (figure 3.41b).

3. Inhaling, straighten your right leg back into three-legged downward-facing dog pose.

(continued)

4. Exhaling, shift forward to plank pose as you pull your right knee toward your left triceps (figure 3.41c).

5. Inhaling, push back to three-legged downward-facing dog pose.

6. Exhaling, shift forward to plank pose as you pull your right knee to your chest and your nose toward your knee, squeezing both the knee and the nose toward each other (figure 3.41d).

7. Inhaling, straighten the leg as you extend back to three-legged downward-facing dog pose.

8. Exhaling, lower the right leg to downward-facing dog pose.

9. Repeat the sequence with the left leg.

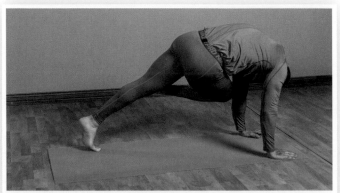

FIGURE 3.41c

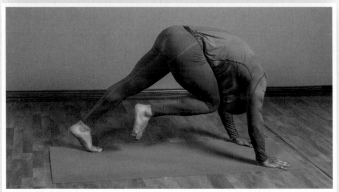

FIGURE 3.41d

Modification

Hold plank pose for 15 to 20 breaths. This variation will build heat in the body and build strength in the core and upper body.

Safety Tips

Stay strong in your core through this movement so that you do not feel any discomfort in your back. If you feel discomfort, follow the modification.

Advanced Flow

Once you are comfortable doing the Sun Salutations with variations, you can put it all together in an advanced flow. The following example includes all the strength-building variations. Remember to breathe! All of these moves should flow on the whispered inhales and exhales of the ujjayi breathing that ties together the breath, blood flow, and exertion.

1 Start by doing two to four repetitions of sun salutation A. Do one regular sun salutation B. On the second sun salutation B, when you step back to plank (figure 3.42), add the double four-limbed staff pose (figure 3.43), then immediately move to holding a side plank on each side (figure 3.44) for 2 to 5 breaths.

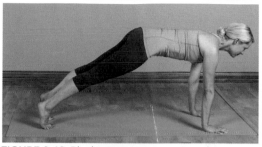

FIGURE 3.42 Plank pose.

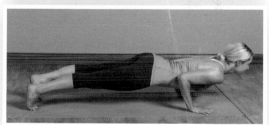

FIGURE 3.43 Four-limbed staff pose.

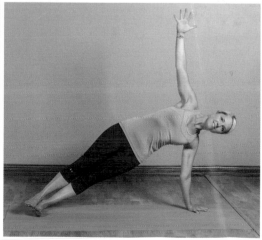

FIGURE 3.44 Side plank.

(continued)

2 Run through another four-limbed staff pose (figure 3.45) to upward-facing dog pose (figure 3.46) and to downward-facing dog pose (figure 3.47).

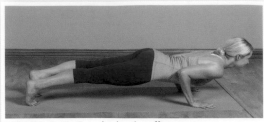

FIGURE 3.45 Four-limbed staff pose.

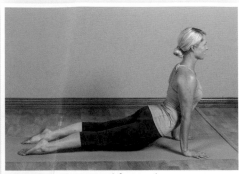

FIGURE 3.46 Upward-facing dog pose.

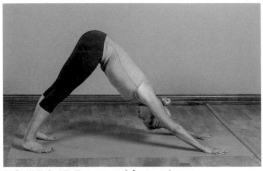

FIGURE 3.47 Downward-facing dog pose.

3 Inhaling, lift your right leg high to the ceiling for three-legged downward-facing dog pose with core work (figure 3.48).

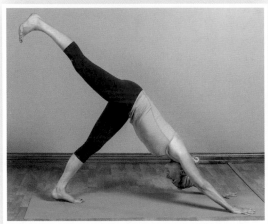

FIGURE 3.48 Three-legged downward-facing dog pose with core work.

4 Exhaling, bring the knee to the right triceps (figure 3.49).

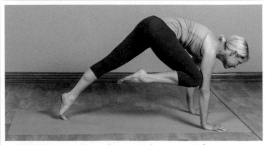

FIGURE 3.49 Three-legged downward-facing dog pose, knee to right triceps.

5 Inhaling, move back up to three-legged downward-facing dog pose. Exhaling, bring the knee to the left triceps (figure 3.50).

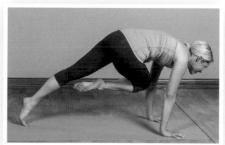

FIGURE 3.50 Three-legged downward-facing dog, knee to left triceps.

6 Inhaling, move back up to three-legged downward-facing dog pose. Exhaling, bring the knee to your nose (figure 3.51).

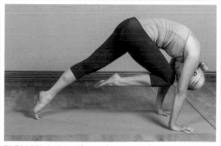

FIGURE 3.51 Three-legged downward-facing dog pose, knee to nose.

7 Inhaling, bring the leg back up to three-legged downward-facing dog. Exhaling, step the right foot forward behind your right wrist and lower the left heel for warrior I pose. Inhaling, lift your arms and torso to complete warrior I pose (figure 3.52).

8 Repeat the sequence with the left leg. Do two more rounds of this sequence to build heat in your body and keep the muscles warm and flexible, completing the variation on sun salutation B.

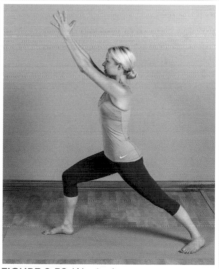

FIGURE 3.52 Warrior I pose.

Summary

This chapter provided a flow of sun salutations to warm you up. Now that you are fully warmed up and feeling strong, it is time to move to the stretches for the various muscles and joints. You can read the chapters individually to learn how to perform each of the stretches, or you can move to part III to see which stretches are most appropriate for your sport, then go back to part II to learn the proper form and technique for each stretch.

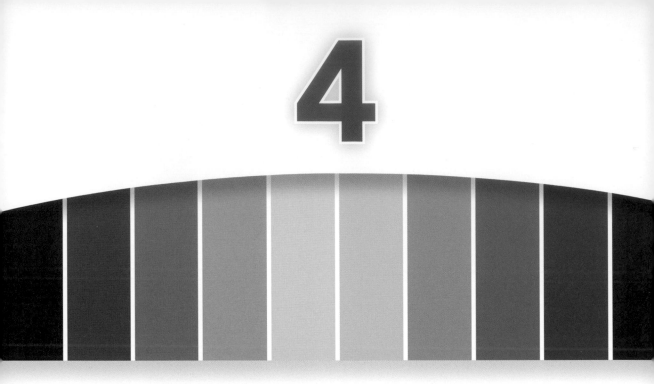

FINDING YOUR BASE: HIPS

The mobility of your hips is important in sports and activities for many reasons. Having full range of motion in your hips helps to enhance your performance, decrease injury, and allow for smooth, fluid movements. Range of motion will increase speed and the quick, short bursts of movement required in any sport. Staying loose in your hips can also alleviate tightness in the low back and even the hamstrings.

Contrary to what many people think, the hips are not only the sides of the body; you should view them as circling around the body's full circumference. The muscles of the outer hips are called your abductors. The muscles at the back of your pelvic area are your gluteal muscles, while the muscles on the front of your pelvis are your hip flexors. The muscles of your inner thighs are the adductors. If the focus of your stretching is on one area of your hips and other areas are neglected, the neglected areas will become increasingly tight. A tight muscle decreases the range of motion in a joint, and in turn this decreased range of motion causes the muscle fibers to shrink, decreasing the muscle's length. All of this tightness creates a pull that leads to misalignment of joints, bones, and eventually overall posture. When this imbalance occurs, a shift in the pelvis known as a pelvic tilt may occur. Tilting the pelvis can lead to low-back problems. Therefore, you should make sure that you stretch all areas of your hips. The hips are the base of your body's alignment and are part of the body's core, also appropriately called the powerhouse. To be successful in your sport, you must take care of your powerhouse.

MATT GUNVILLE

Owner of CrossFit 920, Speed and Power Specialist, Powerlifter

After being a competitive athlete for 20+ years and competing in powerlifting and various strength events, I have dealt with numerous aches and pains. This included a back surgery for herniated disk of my L4 and L5. After doing lots of research and watching my lifting mechanics closely I realized I had an anterior pelvic tilt, more than likely due to tight hamstrings, piriformis, hip flexors, and poor hip mobility. All of these things happening with my mechanics caused most of my injuries. This is where yoga came into play for me. I don't have the enthusiasm for yoga as I do for working out, so I hired Ryanne Cunningham as my professional yoga instructor for help. Take my advice; yoga is well worth it! Stretching out tight muscles and strengthening the weak ones will help with pelvic tilt tremendously. So, this is what Ryanne and I worked on. We started on doing a few certain exercises that focused on opening up my hips, strengthening my core and glutes, and worked on loosening up my prime movers. My back pain wasn't from weak back muscles; it was from poor mobility—a hard lesson to learn. Your body works together like a chain. When one link goes bad, the chain breaks, causing lots of problems. With back pain—or any pain for that matter—we tend to forget that our body works as a whole and that certain antagonists can either be direct or indirect. My advice would be to watch your biomechanics closely, decide where your issues are, and address them with a professional yoga instructor. The benefits I have seen from yoga are faster recovery between workouts, prolonged competitive lifestyle, less warm-up times before lifts, and fewer overall aches and pains.

Happy Baby Pose

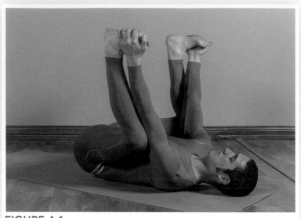

FIGURE 4.1

Muscles

Gluteus maximus, hamstrings, deltoids, biceps

1. Lie on your back.
2. Pull both knees to your chest.
3. Separate the knees, place your arms inside both legs, and reach over the tops of the ankle bones to grab the outer edges of both feet.
4. Separate the feet shoulder-width apart, the bottoms of your feet facing the ceiling.
5. Pull the feet down from the outer edges of both feet, taking your knees toward the floor on the outsides of both shoulders (figure 4.1).
6. Push your tailbone down to the ground.
7. Push your shoulders down to the ground.
8. Puff your chest up.

Modification

Do half happy baby pose with or without the use of a strap.

Safety Tip

Stay away from any knee pain by bending your knee more to decrease any discomfort.

Low Lunging Half Pigeon Pose

Muscles

Hip flexors, upper quadriceps, hamstrings, gluteus maximus, gluteus medius, sartorius, gracilis

1. Start from downward-facing dog pose.
2. Step the right foot forward between the hands.
3. Lower the back knee to the floor.
4. Place both hands on the floor on the inside of the right foot.
5. Turn your right foot to the right slightly so the knee and toes point in the same direction.
6. Flex the right toes up, leaving the ball of the foot down.
7. Gently relax your right knee to the right, rolling to the outer edge of the right foot until you feel the stretch (figure 4.2).
8. Keep your hips in the lunge for a greater stretch.
9. Repeat the pose on the other side.

Modifications

To make this pose easier on especially tight hips, place your hands on a block to keep the torso higher (figure 4.3a) or do not relax the knee to the side (figure 4.3b). For a deeper stretch, place your forearms on a block or the floor and keep lengthening your spine forward.

Safety Tip

If you have knee problems, stay in the low lunge without relaxing the knee to the side. For sensitive knees, place a blanket under your back knee.

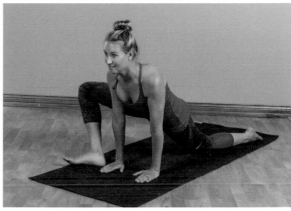

FIGURE 4.2

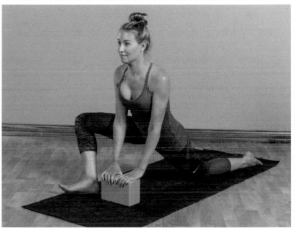

FIGURE 4.3a Low lunging half pigeon pose, modification with block.

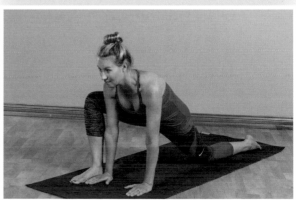

FIGURE 4.3b Low lunging half pigeon pose, modification without block.

Pigeon Pose

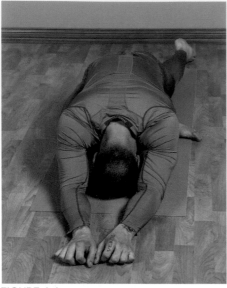

FIGURE 4.4

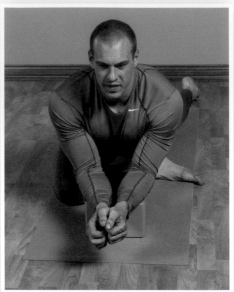

FIGURE 4.5 Pigeon pose, modification with block.

Muscles

Gluteus maximus, gluteus medius, piriformis, sartorius, gracilis, tensor fasciae latae

1. Starting in downward-facing dog pose, bring your right knee to your chest.
2. Place your right knee on the mat, behind your right wrist.
3. Slide your right foot up toward your left hand.
4. Lengthen your left leg back behind you on the mat.
5. Shift your hips back as you square your hips to the front of the mat.
6. Look over your left shoulder, and make sure your left leg is behind your left hip.
7. Lower your forearms to the floor.
8. Extend both arms forward, palms to the floor, and relax your forehead toward or onto the mat (figure 4.4).
9. Keep your hips squared to the front of the mat, and sink your hips down toward the floor.
10. Hold for 10 to 20 breaths.
11. Slowly lift your chest back up, and plant your hands on your mat as you return to downward-facing dog pose.
12. Repeat the pose on the other side.

Modification

Place the bent knee between the hands, keeping the foot by the hips. Place a block under your forearms instead of going all the way down to the floor (figure 4.5).

Safety Tip

Stay away from knee pain in the pose. If pain does occur, come out of this pose immediately and come down to your back for eye of the needle pose.

Eye of the Needle Pose

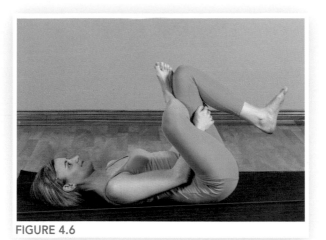

FIGURE 4.6

Muscles

Tensor fasciae latae, gluteus medius, gluteus maximus, piriformis

1. Lie on your back with your knees bent and your feet on the floor.
2. Pull your right knee to your chest.
3. Flex your right foot, and place your right ankle on your left quadriceps, just under the knee.
4. Lift the left foot off the floor.
5. Bend your left knee, and wrap both hands around your left shinbone or hamstrings (figure 4.6).
6. Pull the left leg as close to your chest as possible while pressing the knee open.
7. Repeat the pose on the other side.

Modifications

Wrap both hands around your hamstrings instead of the shinbone, and gently pull the left leg to your chest. If you experience knee pain, plant your left foot back down and maintain the right ankle on the left thigh.

Safety Tip

Watch for any knee discomfort while pulling the left leg to your chest.

Frog Pose

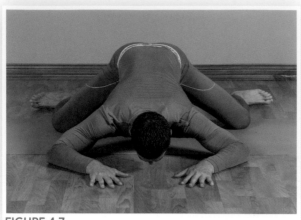

FIGURE 4.7

Muscles

Gracilis, sartorius, adductor brevis, adductor longus, pectineus, adductor magnus

1. Start on your hands and knees.
2. Separate your knees as wide apart as you can.
3. Flex your feet, allowing your toes to point away from each other.
4. Align your legs to a 90-degree angle.
5. Lower your chest to the floor.
6. If necessary, place a block under your breastbone, and rest your chest on it.
7. Rest your forehead on the floor (figure 4.7).
8. Relax your hip joints as your pelvis releases down toward the floor.
9. Hold for 10 to 20 breaths.

Modification

To eliminate pressure on the knees, come to a seat and do bound angle pose.

Safety Tip

This pose is an intense stretch, so be mindful not to overstretch. Also, avoid pain in the knees. If you experience knee pain, move into child's pose.

Revolved One-Legged Chair Pose

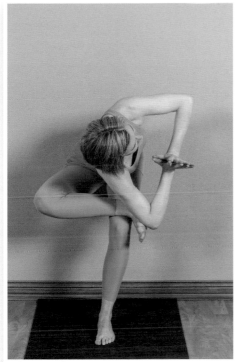

FIGURE 4.8

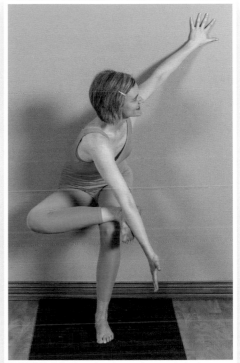

FIGURE 4.9 Revolved one-legged chair pose, modification against a wall.

Muscles

Gluteus maximus, gluteus medius, piriformis, sartorius, gracilis, tensor fasciae latae

1. From a standing position, sit back into chair pose.
2. Place your right ankle on your left thigh, keeping your right foot flexed.
3. Bring your palms together in prayer pose, and place your right elbow on your right inner knee and your left elbow on the arch of your right foot.
4. If you can maintain your balance, twist your torso to the left and place your right elbow onto the arch of your right foot (figure 4.8).
5. Firmly press your palms together to deepen your torso twist to the left. Push your right elbow into your right arch, gently pushing your right foot back behind you.
6. Hold for 5 to 10 breaths.
7. Repeat the pose on the other side.

Modification

Use a wall; lean your hips into the wall and bend your knees. When going into the twist, if your elbow does not meet your arch, place your forearm onto your right arch and your left hand onto the wall (figure 4.9). Push your right forearm into your right arch, and push your foot back behind you. The left hand can rest on the wall for stability.

Rock the Baby Pose

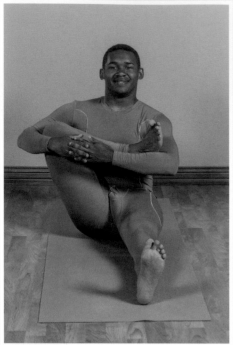

FIGURE 4.10

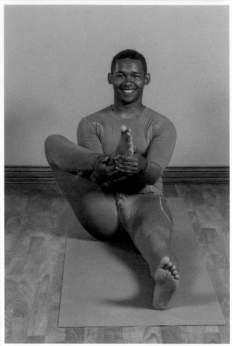

FIGURE 4.11 Rock the baby pose modification.

Muscles

Gluteus maximus, gluteus medius, piriformis

1. Come to a seated position on your mat.
2. Pull your right knee to your chest.
3. With your right hand, place your right foot into the crease of your left elbow, maintaining flexion in your right foot.
4. Wrap your right arm around your right knee, having the crease of the right elbow around your right knee.
5. Interlace your fingers, and hug your right shinbone to your chest (figure 4.10).
6. Sit tall, and lower your shoulders away from your ears.
7. Slowly start to turn at your waist from right to left, maintaining the hug of your leg.
8. Hold for 10-20 breaths.
9. Repeat the pose on the other side.

Modification

Instead of placing the right foot in the crease of the left elbow, place the right foot in the left hand (figure 4.11). Hug the right shinbone to your chest, then start rocking.

Safety Tip

Watch for any discomfort in your right knee. Keep flexion in the foot, and use the modification when needed.

Wide Squat Pose

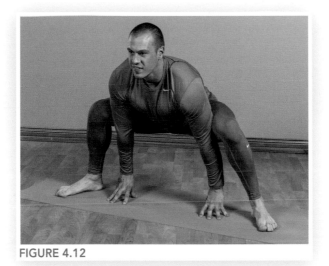

FIGURE 4.12

Muscles

Gastrocnemius, gracilis, adductors, gluteus maximus, quadriceps

1. Stand in the middle of your mat. Separate your feet mat-width apart.
2. Turn your toes out so that they are pointing toward the ends of your mat, and leave your heels on the mat.
3. Bend your knees wide as you lower your hips toward the floor.
4. Place your fingertips or palms to the floor and walk your hands back so your elbows press up onto your inner thighs (figure 4.12).
5. Press your elbows into your inner thighs to push your knees apart. Sink your hips down and lift your chest up.
6. Sink your hips farther down as you lift your chest up to maintain a long torso.
7. Hold for 10 to 20 breaths.

Modifications

This is a deep knee bend, so place a towel behind your knees before going into the squat to allow space in your knees, if needed. Or, try bound angle pose (see figure 4.26). It is a great pose to do in place of the squat. Or place a block under your hips and sit on the block, keeping your elbows on your inner thighs and your palms in prayer to keep the stretch in your inner thighs.

Safety Tip

This pose is a deep bend for the knees, so be careful if you have knee problems.

Plank Pose With IT Band Stretch

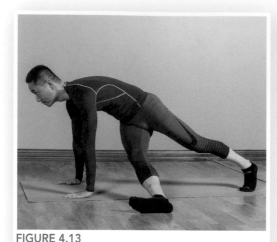

FIGURE 4.13

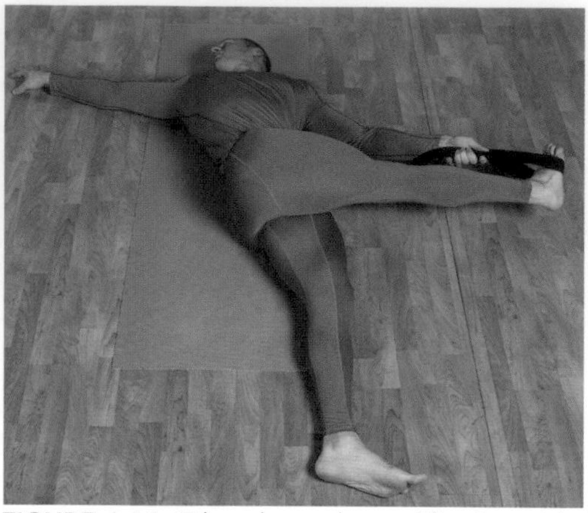

FIGURE 4.14 IT band stretch, modification with back spinal twist.

Muscles

Pectoralis major, deltoids, triceps, serratus anterior, oblique abdominals, rectus abdominis, trapezius, teres major, teres minor, erector spinae, gluteus maximus, gluteus medius, quadriceps, hamstrings, gastrocnemius, tensor fasciae latae, biceps femoris, iliotibial (IT) band

1. Start in plank pose.
2. Bring your right knee toward your chest.
3. Flex your right foot.
4. Straighten your right leg to the left, then place the outer right edge of your foot on the floor off your mat (figure 4.13). Eventually work toward getting your toes to line up with your fingers.
5. Push your left heel back. At the same time, lengthen your collarbones forward and look forward.
6. Keep the arms straight and palms pressing into the floor.
7. Keep flexion in your right foot.
8. Roll your right hip under and back to deepen the stretch.
9. Hold for 5 to 10 breaths.
10. Repeat the pose on the other side.

Modification

Instead of starting in plank pose, lie on your back with your right knee pulled in to your chest and take your leg to the left for a spinal twist (figure 4.14). Straighten your right leg, keeping the right foot flexed.

Safety Tip

Use the modified version of the pose to avoid knee discomfort.

Sage Pose

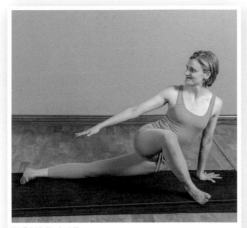

FIGURE 4.15

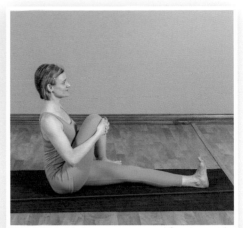

FIGURE 4.16 Sage pose, modification with knee to chest.

Muscles

Gluteus medius, gluteus maximus, tensor fasciae latae

1. From downward-facing dog, step your right foot forward to a low lunge.
2. Place both hands on the mat on the inside of your right foot.
3. Turn your right foot to the right slightly in the same direction your right knee is facing.
4. Curl your back toes under and lift your left knee off the mat slightly as you straighten your back leg out.
5. Put all of your weight onto your left palm.
6. Start to turn to your right by rolling to the outer edge of your back foot and to the outer edge of your right foot, relaxing your right knee to the right.
7. Lower your left hip down toward the floor and reach your arm down along your right side as you gaze down to your left foot (figure 4.15).
8. Hold for 5 to 10 breaths.
9. Repeat the pose on the other side.

Modification

Stay in the seated position, but place your right foot to the outside of the left thigh and hug the knee into the chest with both arms (figure 4.16).

Safety Tip

While on your side, keep a long spine and don't sink into the low back, which may cause discomfort.

Supine Revolving Big Toe Hold With Strap

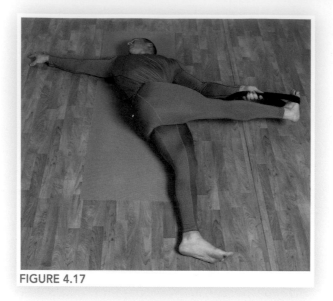

FIGURE 4.17

Muscles

Gluteus medius, tensor fasciae latae, gluteus maximus, piriformis

1. Wrap a strap around your right foot and hold the ends in your left hand. Lying supine (on your back), bring your right knee to your chest.
2. Straighten your right leg up to the ceiling.
3. Reach your right arm down to the floor and off to your right.
4. Slowly lower your right leg toward the floor to your left.
5. Look at your right hand (figure 4.17).
6. Roll your right hip away from your chest to deepen the stretch.

Modification

To make the stretch more advanced, don't use the strap. Instead wrap the left four fingers around the outer edge of your right foot.

Safety Tip

Put a slight bend in your knee to prevent discomfort.

Supine Cow Face Legs

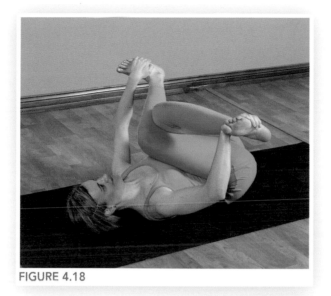

FIGURE 4.18

Muscles

Gluteus medius, gluteus minimus, tensor fasciae latae, piriformis

1. Lie supine (on your back) with both legs bent and the bottoms of your feet on the floor.
2. Cross your right leg completely over your left leg.
3. Lift your feet off your mat.
4. Reach down with both hands for your feet; right hand grabs your left foot, and left hand grabs your right foot.
5. Relax your head down to the mat.
6. Gently pull your knees closer to your chest, then lift your feet up (figure 4.18).
7. Repeat on the other side, left leg crossed over right leg.

Modification

Roll up to a seated position, and bring the bottoms of your feet together for bound angle pose (see figure 4.26).

Safety Tip

If you have tight hips and cannot fully cross your legs, be careful of the pressure on your knees.

Low Lunge Pose With Block

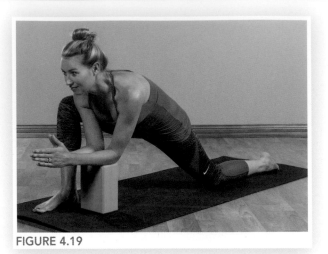

FIGURE 4.19

Muscles

Hip flexors, upper hamstrings, tensor fasciae latae

1. Starting in downward-facing dog pose, step your right foot forward between your hands.
2. Lower your back knee to the floor.
3. Place a block standing tall on the inside of your right foot.
4. Place both hands on your right thigh.
5. Shift your shoulders back so that they are stacked over your hips.
6. Shift your right knee forward, keeping your right ankle under your right knee.
7. Place your hands on the block, staying in the lunge.
8. Lower your forearms to the block.
9. Slide your shoulder down your back, and lengthen your spine forward (figure 4.19).
10. Keep bending your right knee and sinking your hips down to deepen this stretch. You can take the block down to any level you feel comfortable with.
11. Return to downward-facing dog pose, and repeat the pose on the other side.

Modification

Keep your hands on the block.

Safety Tip

To protect the back knee, use a blanket under it as a cushion.

T.W. Side Pigeon Pose

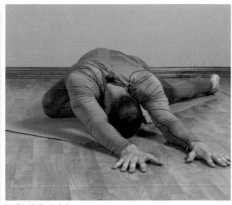

FIGURE 4.20

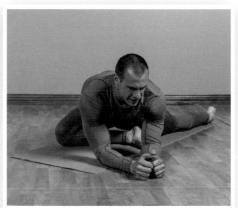

FIGURE 4.21 T.W. side pigeon pose, modification on forearms.

Muscles

Gluteus maximus, gluteus medius, piriformis, tensor fasciae latae

1. Start in pigeon pose (see figure 4.4) with your right knee forward and your head on the mat.
2. Push up so that your forearms are on the floor; your shoulders should align over your elbows.
3. Square your hips to the front of your mat, and start to walk your forearms to the left side of your mat.
4. Extend your right arm out further to the left, and at the same time roll your right hip back and away from you.
5. This stretch has little movement; move your hip forward or back a little until you feel tight and hold that stretch.
6. Once you have found the stretch, relax your head down to the floor and sink your pelvis downward (figure 4.20), holding for 5 to 10 breaths.
7. Lift back up to your forearms, and walk your forearms to the right side of your mat, hovering your chest over your right thigh.
8. Roll your right hip back and forth until you find the hip stretch.
9. Lower your chest to your right thigh, and relax your head to the floor holding for 5 to 10 breaths.
10. Push back to downward-facing dog pose, then move into pigeon pose on the other side. Repeat the sequence on the other side.

Modification

Stay on your forearms (figure 4.21) or come up to your hands to find the hip stretch for both sides. Lower to the forearms only if you do not have any pain or discomfort.

Safety Tip

Make sure to feel this pose only in your hips. If you experience discomfort in your knee, either bend your knee more before going into the side stretch or move your knee to the center of your mat to give your knee plenty of space.

71

Double Pigeon Pose

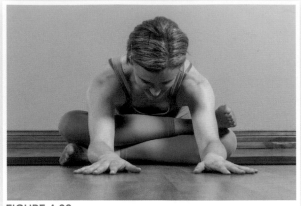

FIGURE 4.22

Muscles

Gluteus maximus, gluteus medius, piriformis, sartorius, gracilis, tensor fasciae latae

1. Begin in a seated position on your mat with your legs stretched out in front of you.
2. Bend your left leg, and lay your leg in front of your hips like a half cross-legged seat.
3. Flexing your right foot, place your right ankle on your left knee.
4. Flexing both feet, slide your left foot up so to be under your right knee.
5. Keep your shins parallel to the front of your mat.
6. Sitting tall, start to lean forward and walk your hands out in front of your legs.
7. Relax your head toward the ground (figure 4.22).
8. Repeat the pose with your left leg on top.

Modifications

While in double pigeon pose with your right knee lifted, place a yoga block between the right knee and left ankle for support (figure 4.23a). Start out with both hands behind your hips, and slowly walk your hands forward until you feel the stretch. If your head doesn't quite make it to the floor, place a yoga block under your forehead and relax your head down (figure 4.23b).

Safety Tip

If you have knee problems, use the modifications to minimize pain or, if this pose is too intense, go into bound angle pose (see figure 4.26).

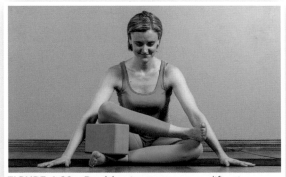

FIGURE 4.23a Double pigeon pose, modification with a block between the knees.

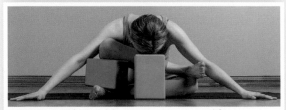

FIGURE 4.23b Double pigeon pose, modification with a block under the forehead.

Seated Cow Face Pose

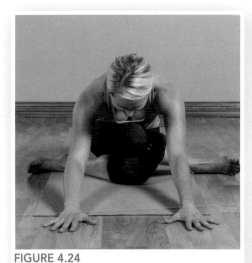

FIGURE 4.24

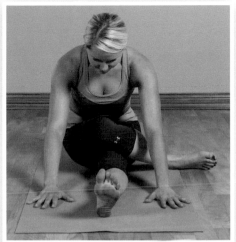

FIGURE 4.25 Seated cow face pose, modification with the bottom leg straight.

Muscles

Piriformis, gluteus maximus, gluteus medius, gluteus minimus, tensor fasciae latae

1. Begin in a seated position on your mat with both legs lengthened in front of you.
2. Bring your right knee to your chest, and cross your right leg over your left leg, stacking your knees.
3. Bend your left leg, sliding your left foot next to your right hip while keeping your knees stacked.
4. Walk your hands forward as you lay your chest on your thighs (figure 4.24).

Modification

If your hips are very tight, keep the bottom leg straight (figure 4.25). This modification makes the hip stretch less intense and more accessible.

Safety Tip

Go into this pose slowly to make sure your knees are comfortable before intensifying it.

Bound Angle Pose

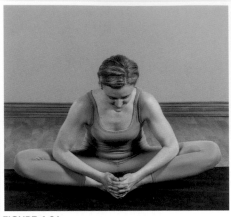

FIGURE 4.26

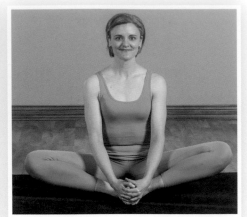

FIGURE 4.27 Bound angle pose, modification with the torso remaining upright.

Muscles

Gluteus medius, gluteus minimus, tensor fasciae latae, Adductors

1. Sit on your mat.
2. Bend both knees, and place the soles of your feet together as you relax your knees down to your sides.
3. Place your hands around your feet, and lean your upper body forward (figure 4.26).

Modifications

If you feel discomfort in the knees or back, don't lean forward; instead, sit tall (figure 4.27).

Summary

The hips are more than areas at the sides of the body; they are the power-house of energy in any sport or workout. Apply any of the hip stretches in this chapter to your training routine. Athletes need to stay injury free and keep their bodies as healthy as possible. Taking the time pre- and post-workout or training to stretch the hips can increase your power in your sport.

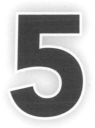

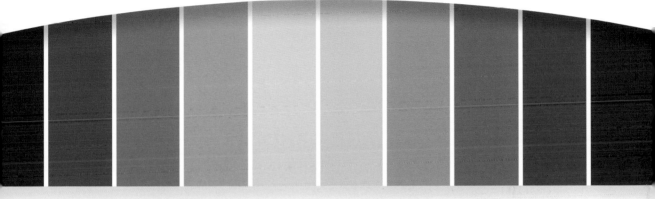

STAYING LOOSE IN THE LEGS: HAMSTRINGS AND QUADRICEPS

The hamstrings and quadriceps are the two major muscle groups of the upper leg. The origin of the hamstring muscles is at the tuberosity of the ischium and linea aspera, which attach at the pelvis near your sitting bones. The hamstrings insert at the tibia and fibula behind the knee halfway down the leg. If your hamstrings are tight, they can pull your pelvis out of alignment. This shift in your hips can increase pain in your back, hips, and knees, and it can increase the chances of injury when you participate in a sport. This shift will also limit you in forward folds and some standing poses. Working on the flexibility of your hamstrings can help increase the length of your stride and increase your speed, and it can also can enhance your form for your sport, thus keeping you on the field.

The quadriceps are powerful, complex, hard-working muscles that are used in almost all sports. People tend to neglect the quadriceps in yoga practice and seldom stretch them after workouts. The origin of the quadriceps is the rectus femoris and vastus muscles, while the quadriceps insertion is the tibial tuberosity. In many sports, the quadriceps are stretched before an event but little after the event. Tight quadriceps can greatly affect the knees, spine, and hips. In certain sports the quadriceps are used often, and in yoga they assist in stretching the hamstrings while in seated or standing poses.

AMANDA RHODES
Edgewood College Soccer

As an athlete, yoga has been amazing not only for my recovery, but also for the health of my mind and muscles. In soccer you are focused on the game, anticipation of plays, and strategy, as well as exerting yourself for long periods of time. During 90 minutes of play the average soccer player will run 5 to 7 miles. This amount of strenuous activity paired with a game of anticipation requires taking care of your body and mind. Your hamstrings get tight from all the running, your quads are burning from ball handling and shooting, and your ankles and calves are tight from playing on an uneven surface when on a grass field. Yoga is amazing because it quiets your mind before a game; it relaxes and connects to your body before entering the pitch. The practice of yoga itself is beneficial for building strength and endurance in both large and small supportive muscle groups and, what I feel is most important . . . promotes flexibility with all of our muscle groups to allow for improved muscle development and less injury.

Pyramid Pose With Block

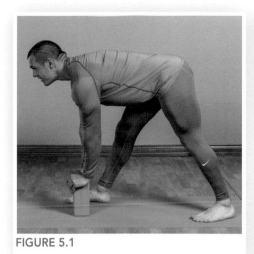

FIGURE 5.1

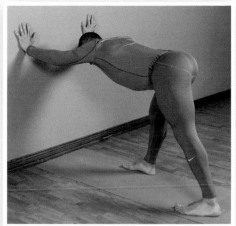

FIGURE 5.2 Pyramid pose, modification with a wall.

Muscles

Hamstrings (semitendinosus, biceps femoris, semimembranosus)

1. Start in downward-facing dog pose. Bring your right knee to your chest, then plant your right foot behind your right hand.
2. Hop your left foot forward until you can angle the back heel down and both feet are flat on the ground (usually about 6 inches, or 15 cm).
3. Place a yoga block standing tall next to the inside of the front foot.
4. Come up to standing, and square your hips to the front of the mat, lengthening the torso forward.
5. Place both hands on the block (figure 5.1).
6. Press the ball of your right foot firmly down.
7. Push your right hip back a bit farther.
8. Lift and lengthen your collarbones forward.
9. Draw in your belly slightly.
10. Push your back foot down evenly onto your mat.
11. If you can go deeper into this hamstring stretch, take your block down a level or two or place your hands on the floor.
12. Hold the pose for 15 to 20 breaths.
13. Move back to downward-facing dog pose, then repeat the pose on the left side.

Modification

Use a wall. Facing a wall, start the same way with the legs. Instead of lowering down to a block, place your palms on the wall (figure 5.2). Slide your shoulders down away from your ears. Square your hips, and breathe.

Safety Tip

Do not hyperextend the knees or overstretch the hamstrings. Ease into this pose, taking each step slowly.

Reclining Hand to Big Toe Pose

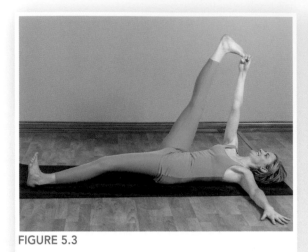

FIGURE 5.3

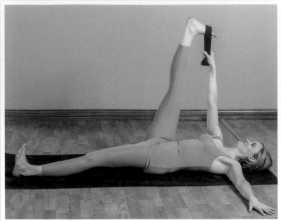

FIGURE 5.4 Reclining hand to big toe pose, modification with strap.

Muscles

Hamstrings (semitendinosus, biceps femoris, semimembranosus)

1. Lying on your back, bring your right knee into your chest. Keep your left leg straight on the floor.
2. Hook your pointer and middle finger between your big toe and second toe, wrapping your fingers around the big toe.
3. Keep your head on the floor.
4. Straighten your right leg up to the ceiling as you push through your heel (figure 5.3).
5. Keeping your leg straight, slowly pull your leg closer to your chest for a deeper stretch.
6. Hold the pose for 5 to 10 breaths, and repeat on the other side.

Modification

Place a strap around the ball of your foot (figure 5.4). You can also hold the strap with each hand. To deepen this stretch, keep walking the hands up the strap toward the foot.

Safety Tip

Watch for hyperextension in the knee, which can cause discomfort or pain. Maintain a microbend in your knee if needed.

Wide-Legged Forward Fold

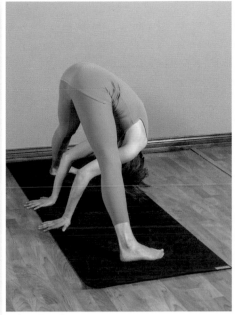

FIGURE 5.5

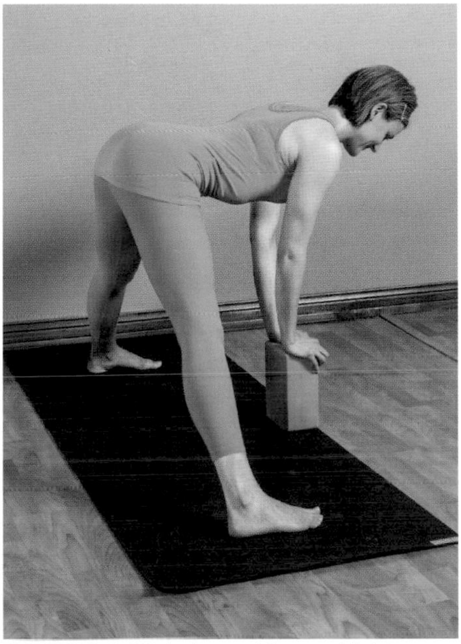

FIGURE 5.6 Wide-legged forward fold, modification with a block.

Muscles

Hamstrings (semitendinosus, biceps femoris, semimembranosus)

1. Stand at the top of your mat.
2. Take a big step back with your left foot.
3. Turn both feet to the left so that both feet face the same direction and are parallel to each other.
4. Place your hands on your hips.
5. Bend both knees, and hinge at your hips as you lower your torso toward the floor.
6. Place your palms on the mat.
7. Turn your hands around so that your fingers point behind you (figure 5.5).
8. Press your palms down into the mat so that you can lengthen the top of your head to the mat.
9. Straighten your legs as you keep lifting your hips up to the ceiling.
10. Hold the stretch for 10 to 15 breaths.

Modification

Place a block on your mat, standing tall. Place both hands on the block (figure 5.6). Keep a long spine forward; do not hunch forward toward the floor. Straighten your legs.

Safety Tip

Maintain a microbend in both knees to prevent hyperextension. Keep your core slightly engaged to protect your low back.

Half Squat Pose

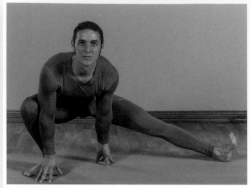

FIGURE 5.7

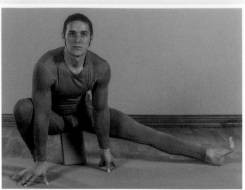

FIGURE 5.8 Half squat pose, modification with a block.

Muscles

Hamstrings (semitendinosus, biceps femoris, semimembranosus)

1. From a wide-legged forward fold, place your hands on the mat under your chest.
2. Turn both feet out slightly so that your toes point away from you. Make sure your toes and knees point in the same direction.
3. Bend your right knee, and walk your hands to the right foot, taking your right knee over your right ankle.
4. As you bend your right knee, straighten your left leg.
5. Flex the left foot so that the toes point up toward the ceiling.
6. Sink your hips and lift your chest, using your hands for stability as needed (figure 5.7).
7. The right arm can gently push into the right thigh to deepen the stretch.
8. The right heel can be on the floor or lifted off the floor.
9. Hold the pose for 5 to 10 breaths, then repeat on the other side.

Modifications

Lift your right heel high as you bend your right knee. Go only halfway to the right until you feel the stretch in your left leg. You may also place a block under your hips and sit on the block (figure 5.8).

Safety Tip

While in any variation of this pose, make sure to feel the stretch in the hamstrings, not the inner knee. You should not feel any knee discomfort. If you feel discomfort in the knee, slowly rotate the leg externally or internally to get out of the discomfort. You may also plant the left foot on the floor.

Seated Forward Fold

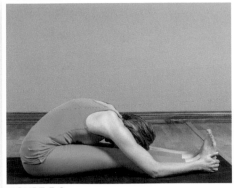

FIGURE 5.9

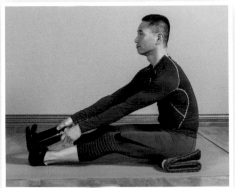

FIGURE 5.10 Seated forward fold, modification with a blanket and strap.

Muscles

Hamstrings (semitendinosus, biceps femoris, semimembranosus)

1. Sit on your mat with both legs straight in front of you.
2. Rotate the legs in toward each together, and flex your feet so that the toes point toward the ceiling.
3. Sitting up tall, reach both arms toward the ceiling.
4. Hinging at your hips, reach forward for your toes.
5. Wrap your hands around your feet. For a deeper stretch, you can relax your head down to your shins (figure 5.9).
6. Hold the stretch for 10 to 20 breaths.

Modification

Sit on a blanket. Keep a slight bend in both knees. Wrap a strap around your feet, and walk your hands down the strap until you feel a stretch in your hamstrings (figure 5.10).

Safety Tip

Keep your core slightly engaged to protect your low back. If you feel an intense stretch in your low back, ease up a bit. Focus on the hamstring stretch.

Triangle Pose

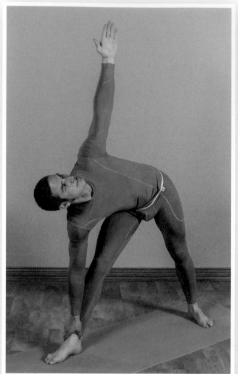

FIGURE 5.11

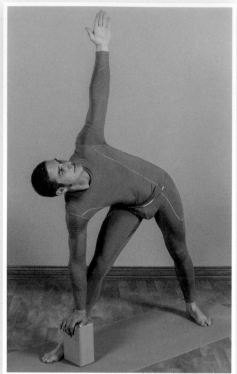

FIGURE 5.12 Triangle pose, modification with a block.

Muscles

Hamstrings (semitendinosus, biceps femoris, semimembranosus)

1. Start in downward-facing dog pose. Step your right foot forward between your hands.
2. Turn your back heel down, and lift your torso to standing.
3. Your feet should be about one leg length apart with your front heel in line with your back arch.
4. Keep your legs straight as you reach your right arm forward in front of you.
5. Lean your upper body forward, keeping your spine long with no rounding. Push your right hip back.
6. Once you feel the stretch, relax your right hand down to your shin or the floor.
7. Reach your left arm up to the ceiling, stacking your shoulders (figure 5.11).
8. Lengthen your tailbone down toward your left heel, and lengthen your spine forward.
9. Hold the pose for 5 to 10 breaths, and repeat on the other side.

Modification

Place a block on either side of the front leg, and place your hand on top of the block. (figure 5.12).

Safety Tip

Maintain a long spine. Do not round the back, which can cause back pain.

Crossed Ankles Forward Fold

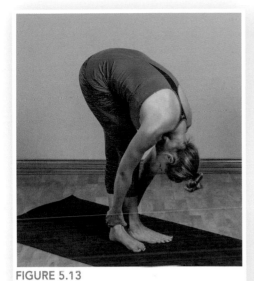

FIGURE 5.13

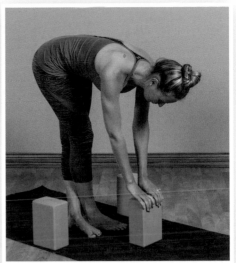

FIGURE 5.14 Crossed ankles forward fold, modification with blocks.

Muscles

Hamstrings (semitendinosus, biceps femoris, semimembranosus)

1. Stand at the top of your mat.
2. Cross your right foot over your left, and plant your right foot on the floor.
3. Turn your heels into each other so that your toes fan away from each other.
4. Press firmly onto the balls of both big toes, making sure the outer heels stay on the mat.
5. Bend both knees and fold forward, placing both hands on the floor in front of your feet.
6. Straighten both legs; the front knee will have a slight bend.
7. Keep pushing both feet firmly into the floor.
8. Stay in the forward fold and walk your hands to your right. Lengthen your left hand out for a deeper stretch.
9. Walk your hands to the left side of your mat. Lengthen your hand out for a deeper stretch.
10. Walk your hands back to the center.
11. Fold forward, and try to wrap one or both hands around your ankles to challenge your balance (figure 5.13).
12. Hold the stretch for 5 to 10 breaths, and repeat it on the other side.

Modification

Use blocks if not able to touch the ground (figure 5.14).

Variation: Twisted Flat Back

Stand at the top of your mat with your feet hip-width apart. Deeply bend both knees, and fold forward. Hook four fingers of your left hand under the outer edge of your

(continued)

right foot and place your right palm on your low back. Lengthen your torso through your collarbones to a twisted flat back position. Keep the left arm straight, and straighten the right leg to keep your left knee bent. Twist your right shoulder back. For a deeper stretch, lean your upper back away as you twist to the right. Hold the pose for 5 to 10 breaths and repeat it on the other side.

If you have loose hamstrings, straighten both legs while in the twist. If you are struggling to hook your fingers under your foot, wrap your hand around your outer leg or place a yoga block to the outside of your foot.

Safety Tip

Hyperextension can easily happen in this pose. Watch out for hyperextension, and maintain a microbend in both knees if needed.

Runner's Back Lunge Pose

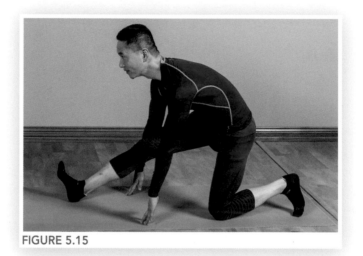

FIGURE 5.15

Muscles

Hamstrings (semitendinosus, biceps femoris, semimembranosus)

1. From downward-facing dog pose, step your right foot forward and lower your left knee to the ground.
2. Place both hands on your right thigh, and bend your right knee forward, sinking your left hip forward and down, making sure your right ankle is under your right knee.
3. Bring your hands down to the floor; the right hand is on the outside of the right leg, and the left hand is on the inside of your right leg.
4. Curl your left toes under, and shift your hips back toward your left foot as you straighten your right leg. Your hips will not touch your left heel; they will be high.
5. Flex your right foot so that your toes point up (figure 5.15).

6. Walk your hands toward your right foot, and lower your head until you find your hamstring stretch.

7. Hold the pose for 5 to 15 breaths, and repeat on the other side.

Modification

If your hamstrings are very tight, use a block either on the inside or outside of your right leg to elevate your torso.

Safety Tip

This pose may cause discomfort in the back knee. If so, place a blanket under your knee to cushion it.

Seated Wide-Legged Forward Fold

Muscles

Hamstrings (semitendinosus, biceps femoris, semimembranosus)

1. Sit on your mat with both legs forward and wide apart.

2. Flex the feet to point the toes to the ceiling.

3. Sit tall with the hands on the floor behind your hips, pressing into the floor.

4. Bring your hands in front of your hips, and walk the hands out as your try to lower to your forearms and then to your forehead (figure 5.16). Go only as far as you feel the stretch. Hold it for 10 to 20 breaths.

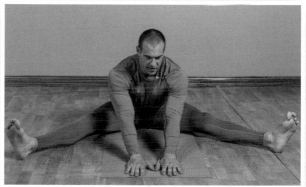

FIGURE 5.16

Modifications

For some people, sitting up tall is enough of a stretch or put your hands on the blocks for a deeper stretch (figure 5.17). You can place the blocks behind your hips. If your forearms or head do not reach the floor, you can place a block in front of your hips to elevate the floor.

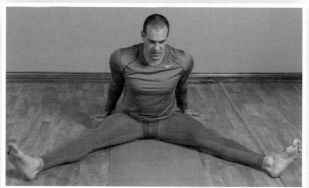

FIGURE 5.17 Seated wide-legged forward fold, modification with blocks

Safety Tip

To help you stay in the hamstring stretch and avoid discomfort in the inner knee, keep your feet flexed and your toes reaching upward.

Revolved Head to Knee Pose

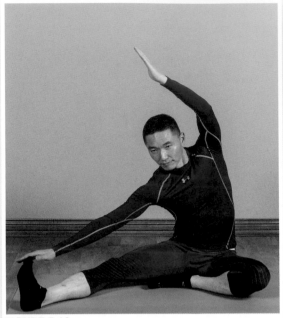

FIGURE 5.18

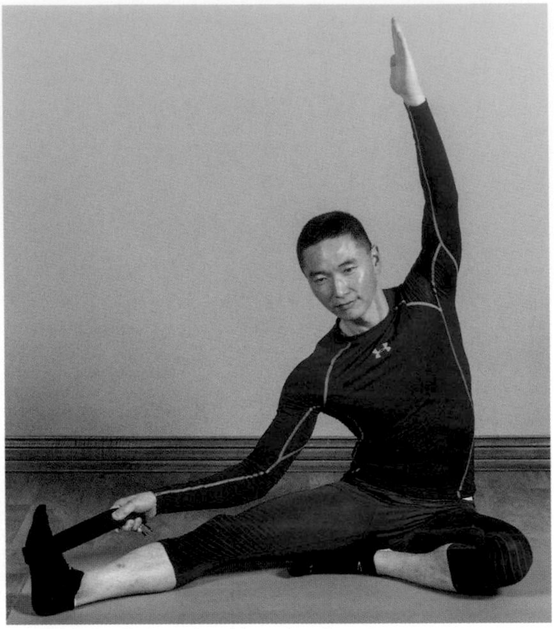

FIGURE 5.19 Revolved head to knee pose, modification with a strap.

Muscles

Hamstrings (semitendinosus, biceps femoris, semimembranosus)

1. Sit with your legs wide. Bend your left knee, and place the bottom of the left foot against the inner thigh of your right leg.
2. Lower your right arm to the inside of your right leg, and take hold of your right foot.
3. Roll your left shoulder back and lengthen your left arm overhead, taking hold of your right foot as you revolve the chest toward the ceiling (figure 5.18).
4. Hold the pose for 5 to 10 breaths, and repeat it on the other side.

Modification

Wrap a strap around your right foot (figure 5.19). Reach your right hand as far down the strap as you can. Hold the strap. Roll your left shoulder back, and reach your left arm overhead.

Safety Tip

This pose sometimes bothers the shoulders. Instead of reaching the top arm overhead, wrap it behind your back or let it rest at your side.

Head to Knee Pose

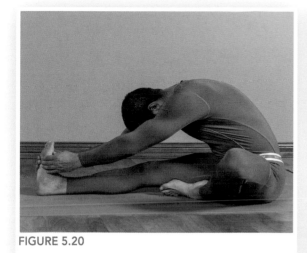

FIGURE 5.20

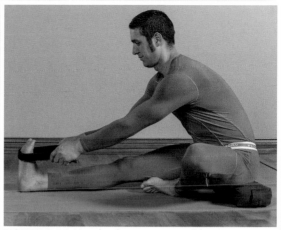

FIGURE 5.21 Head to knee pose, modification on a bolster and with a strap.

Muscles

Hamstrings (semitendinosus, biceps femoris, semimembranosus)

1. Begin in a seated position with both legs stretched out in front of you.
2. Bring your left knee up to your chest, and plant the left foot on the floor on the inside of your right thigh.
3. Lower your left knee toward the floor.
4. Sit tall as you reach both arms up to the ceiling and fold forward, taking hold of your right foot with both hands.
5. Keep your shoulders back and your spine long as you relax your head down to your right leg (figure 5.20).
6. Hold the stretch for 5 to 10 breaths, then repeat it on the other side.

Modification

If your hamstrings are tight, sit on a blanket or bolster to help lift the hips higher. Use a strap around your right foot to help you in the stretch so that you can slowly work your way to the foot (figure 5.21).

Safety Tip

Tight hamstrings may cause back discomfort, so go slowly in this pose to prevent back pain or pulling of any muscles.

Low Lunge Pose

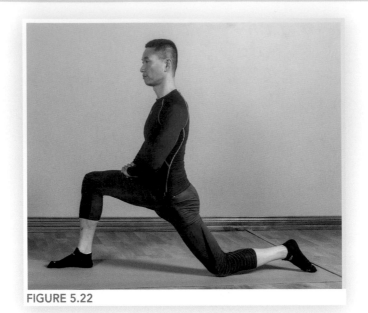

FIGURE 5.22

Muscles

Quadriceps (rectus femoris, vastus lateralis, vastus intermedius, vastus medialis)

1. Start in downward-facing dog pose. Step your right foot forward between your hands.
2. Lower your left knee to the floor.
3. Place both hands on your right thigh.
4. Shift your shoulders back over your hips as you lengthen up through the torso.
5. Bend your right knee forward, keeping your right ankle under your right knee.
6. Shift your hips and left thigh forward and down toward the ground (figure 5.22).
7. Hold the pose for 10 to 15 breaths, then repeat it on the other side.

Modification

Instead of sinking forward into the lunge, stay high and hold here to slowly work into the full low lunge pose.

Safety Tip

Place a blanket under the back knee to cushion and protect the knee.

Low Lunge Pose Variation

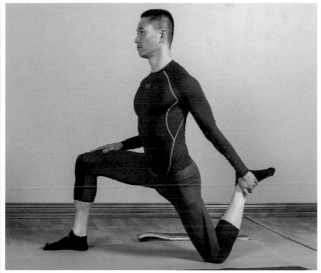

FIGURE 5.23

Muscles

Quadriceps (rectus femoris, vastus lateralis, vastus intermedius, vastus medialis)

1. Start in low lunge pose with the right leg forward and the left knee on the mat.
2. Shift your hips back so that they are over the left knee.
3. Reach back with your left hand as you lift your left foot off the mat and toward the ceiling.
4. Take hold of the outside of the left foot.
5. Bend your right knee forward, and move back into the low lunge (figure 5.23).
6. Keep your left arm straight as you square your shoulders toward the front of your mat.
7. If it's comfortable, bend your left elbow and point it toward the ceiling as you pull your left heel toward your left hip.
8. Hold the pose for 5 to 10 breaths, then repeat it on the other side.

Modifications

If you have difficulty grabbing the back foot, loop a strap around the foot. Also, to help with balance, place a block on the inside or outside of your front leg and rest your front hand on it (figure 5.24).

Safety Tips

Use a blanket to cushion your back knee. While reaching for the back foot, go slowly to prevent any hamstring cramping.

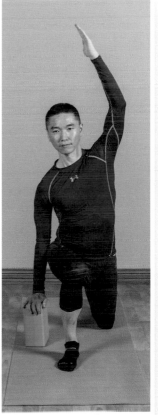

FIGURE 5.24 Low lunge pose variation, modification with a block.

Crescent Lunge Pose

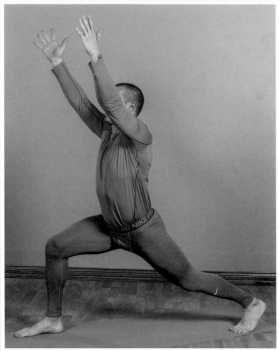

FIGURE 5.25

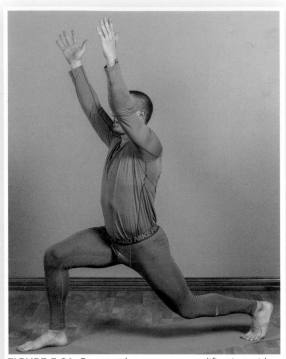

FIGURE 5.26 Crescent lunge pose, modification with the back knee bent.

Muscles

Quadriceps (rectus femoris, vastus lateralis, vastus intermedius, vastus medialis)

1. Start from downward-facing dog pose. Step your right foot forward behind your right hand.
2. Keeping your back knee off the ground press the left heel toward the back of your mat.
3. Lift your torso up until your shoulders are over your hips, and reach both arms toward the ceiling.
4. Keep your front knee over your ankle.
5. Engage the lower belly, dropping your tailbone downward to protect your low back and ensure a long spine.
6. Deepen the bend in your front knee, and push your back heel toward the back of your mat, allowing your hips to sink slightly (figure 5.25).
7. Hold the pose for 5 to 10 breaths, then repeat it on the other side.

Modification

Maintain your crescent lunge pose, but add a bend in your back knee to hover the mat (figure 5.26). Keep your tailbone tucked downward and your lower belly engaged. You should still feel the quadriceps stretch.

Safety Tip

It is easy to feel discomfort in the low back. Keeping the core engaged, tailbone tucking downward, and a bend in the back knee will help to prevent the discomfort.

High Lunge Pose

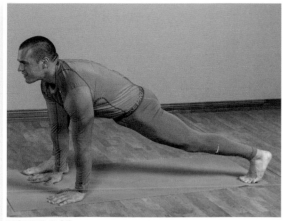

FIGURE 5.27

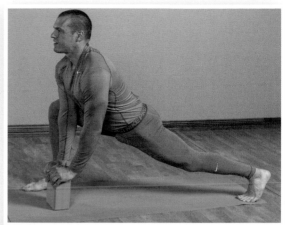

FIGURE 5.28 High lunge pose, modification with a block.

Muscles

Quadriceps (rectus femoris, vastus lateralis, vastus intermedius, vastus medialis)

1. From downward-facing dog pose, step your right foot forward between your hands.
2. Place your right hand on the inside of your right foot.
3. Toe-heel your right foot a few steps to the right to give your shoulders some space.
4. Slide your shoulder blades down your back.
5. Press your palms into your mat, lifting your chest up slightly and keeping your gaze forward.
6. Bend your right knee, and push your left heel back (figure 5.27).
7. Allow your hips to sink downward.
8. Hold the pose for 5 to 10 breaths, then repeat it on the other side.

Modifications

If you cannot reach the ground without rounding your back, place a block standing tall on the inside of your right foot to elevate the ground, and place both hands on the block (figure 5.28). If this pose is too intense, lower the back knee to the floor and practice low lunge pose.

Safety Tips

Enter into this pose slowly so that you are aware enough to avoid overstretching. Be mindful of any knee discomfort, and modify the pose accordingly if needed.

Twisting High Lunge Pose

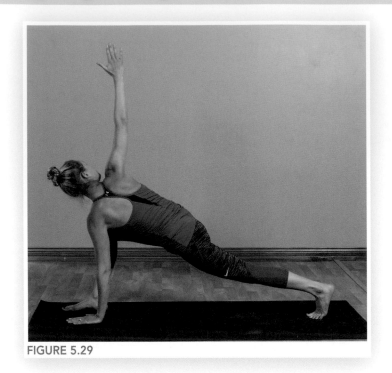

FIGURE 5.29

Muscles

Quadriceps (rectus femoris, vastus lateralis, vastus intermedius, vastus medialis)

1. Step your right foot forward, and begin in high lunge pose.
2. Put your weight into your left palm.
3. Reach your right arm up to the ceiling, twisting your torso to the right (figure 5.29).
4. Bend your right knee forward and push your left heel back at the same time.
5. Sink your left thigh down toward the floor but not all the way to the floor.
6. Hold the pose for 5 to 10 breaths, then repeat it on the other side.

Modifications

Maintain all the steps in your high lunge, twist but lower the back knee to the floor, placing a blanket under the knee for a cushion. Or place a yoga block under your left hand to give your torso elevation.

Safety Tip

Keep your core slightly engaged to prevent any back discomfort.

Wall Stretch

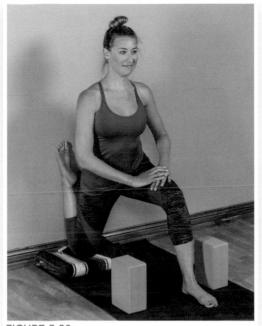

FIGURE 5.30

Muscles

Quadriceps (rectus femoris, vastus lateralis, vastus intermedius, vastus medialis)

1. Place your mat by a wall.
2. Come to your hands and knees facing away from the wall.
3. Lift your right leg behind you, keeping your knee bent, and place your right shinbone on the wall, toe pointing to the ceiling.
4. Slide your right knee down to the floor, leaving just your shin and the top of your foot on the wall.
5. Lift your left knee off the floor, and plant your left foot on the floor.
6. Place both hands on your left thigh as you lift your chest.
7. Slowly push the left foot into the floor, taking your hips and upper body back toward the wall.
8. Once your right hip touches your right heel, shift your hips to the left so that your right heel is on the outside of the right hip.
9. Slowly lean your hips and back toward the wall (figure 5.30).
10. Hold the stretch for 10 to 20 breaths, then repeat it on the other side.

Modification

Cushion your right knee and keep the right knee 1/2 to 1 inch away from the wall. Place two blocks on either side of your left foot for both hands, and stay low if your quadriceps are tight.

Safety Tip

This stretch is intense, so be cautious of any knee discomfort and keep the focus on the quadriceps.

King Pigeon Pose

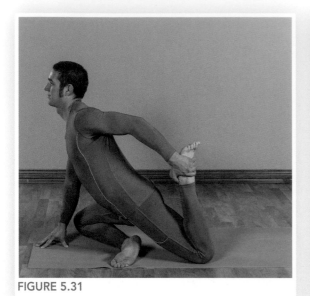

FIGURE 5.31

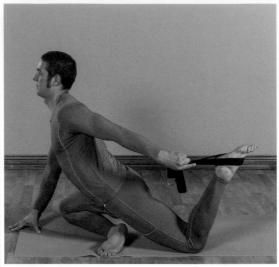

FIGURE 5.32 King pigeon pose, modification with a strap.

Muscles

Quadriceps (rectus femoris, vastus lateralis, vastus intermedius, vastus medialis)

1. Start in downward-facing dog pose. Bend your right knee, drawing it in to your chest.
2. Place your right knee down behind your right wrist.
3. Slide your right foot up toward your left hand.
4. Lengthen your left leg back.
5. Shift your hips back as you square them to the front of your mat.
6. Look over your left shoulder, and make sure your left leg is directly behind your left hip.
7. Bend your left knee, and reach back with your left hand for your foot or ankle.
8. Square your shoulders and hips and look forward, keeping your left arm straight.
9. Bend your left elbow up to the ceiling, and pull your heel closer to your gluteal muscles for a deeper stretch (figure 5.31).
10. Hold the pose for 5 to 10 breaths, then repeat it on the other side.

Modification

If reaching your foot or ankle is impossible, loop a strap around the left foot (figure 5.32).

Safety Tips

Be cautious of any knee discomfort. Instead of placing the knee behind the wrist, place your knee between your hands and keep your foot close to your hips. When reaching back for your left foot before bending the knee, be careful of hamstring cramping. If cramping starts to happen, stop and avoid this part of the stretch by keeping the back leg straight.

Side-Bending Low Lunge Pose

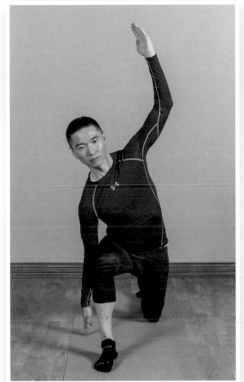

FIGURE 5.33

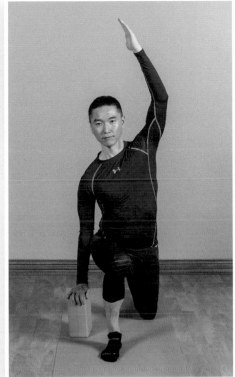

FIGURE 5.34 Side-bending low lunge pose, modification with a block.

Muscles

Quadriceps (rectus femoris, vastus lateralis, vastus intermedius, vastus medialis)

1. From downward-facing dog pose, step your right foot forward and lower your left knee to the floor into a low lunge pose.
2. Lift your torso, aligning your shoulders over your hips, and press your hips forward in your low lunge.
3. Relax your right arm down along your side, and reach your left arm up to the ceiling.
4. Stay in your low lunge as you slowly lean your torso to the right, working your right fingertips toward the ground until they touch (figure 5.33).
5. Move your left shoulder back or forward until you feel the stretch in your left side, then hold the stretch.
6. Keep your torso in line with the hips and not leaning too far forward.
7. Hold the pose for 10 to 15 breaths, then repeat it on the other side.

Modification

Place a yoga block under your right hand to elevate the ground, and slowly work your hand toward the ground (figure 5.34).

Safety Tip

Keep your lower core slightly engaged to protect your back.

One-Legged Frog Pose

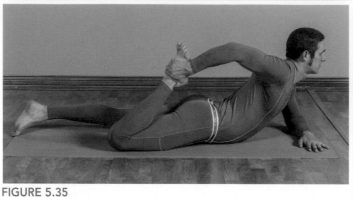

FIGURE 5.35

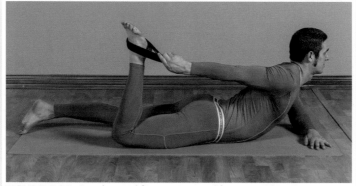

FIGURE 5.36 One-legged frog pose, modification with a strap.

Muscles

Quadriceps (rectus femoris, vastus lateralis, vastus intermedius, vastus medialis)

1. Lie on your belly on your mat.
2. Lift your chest, and place your forearms on the ground, aligning your elbows under your shoulders.
3. Bend your right knee.
4. Circle your right hand around behind you, and place your right hand on the top of your right foot.
5. Bend your right elbow up as you pull your right foot toward your right hip (figure 5.35).
6. Keep your spine long by lengthening your chest forward and your tailbone back.
7. Hold the pose for 5 to 10 breaths, then repeat it on the other side.

Modification

If your quadriceps or shoulders are too tight to reach your foot, loop a strap around your right foot to help to deepen this stretch (figure 5.36).

Safety Tip

Avoid sinking into your low back; maintain core engagement and a long spine.

Reclining Hero Pose

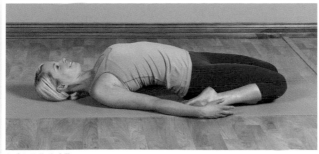

FIGURE 5.37

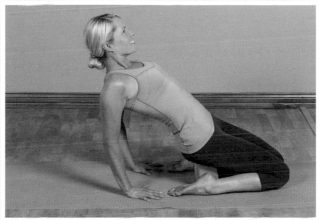

FIGURE 5.38 Hero pose, modification with a block.

Muscles

Quadriceps (rectus femoris, vastus lateralis, vastus intermedius, vastus medialis)

1. Sit on your heels with your shinbones on your mat.
2. Separate your feet hip-width apart, keeping your knees together.
3. Sink your hips down to the floor between your feet.
4. Slowly walk your hands back behind you as you lower down to your back (figure 5.37).
5. Tuck your tailbone toward your knees to lengthen your back and keep your knees together and on the floor.
6. Relax your arms down at your sides.
7. Hold the pose for 10 to 15 breaths.

Modification

Use a yoga block under your hips (figure 5.38) if your quadriceps are tight or you have discomfort in your knees. If you use the block, keep your torso up instead of reclining.

Safety Tip

Watch for any discomfort in your knees and back, and use the modification if this pose is too intense.

Twisting Low Lunge Pose With Quadriceps Stretch

Muscles

Quadriceps (rectus femoris, vastus lateralis, vastus intermedius, vastus medialis)

1. From downward-facing dog pose, step your right foot forward to a low lunge pose.
2. Place both hands to the floor on the inside of your right foot.
3. Maintain a long spine.
4. Put your weight into your left hand, and bend your left knee.
5. Start to twist your torso to the right, circling your right hand around, and clasp your left foot (figure 5.39).
6. Keep your focal point at the back of your mat somewhere to help keep you in the spinal twist.
7. Bend your right knee to shift your hips forward as you pull your left heel closer to your left hip.
8. Hold the pose for 5 to 15 breaths, and repeat it on the other side.

Modification

Use a yoga block under your left hand (figure 5.40) to elevate the ground and lessen the intensity of the stretch on tight quadriceps. The block also allows you to move into the pose slowly and with ease.

Safety Tips

Be easy on your back knee by using a soft blanket or small bolster for support. While in this stretch, keep your back heel and hip in line with each other. It is very easy to pull the back foot toward the opposite hip.

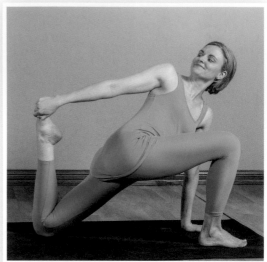

FIGURE 5.39

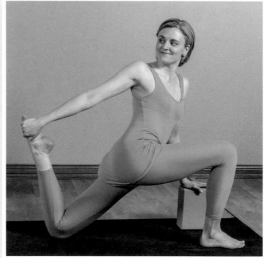

FIGURE 5.40 Twisting low lunge pose with quadriceps stretch, modification with a block.

Summary

This chapter explained the basics of stretching both the hamstrings and quadriceps, the two major muscle groups of the upper leg. The poses in this chapter focus on stretching these muscle groups, which are crucial in every sport and workout. Adding even a few minutes a day of poses related to stretching these areas will benefit your body and your performance.

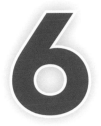

RADIATING STRENGTH FROM THE CENTER: SPINE AND CORE

Having a strong core can help prevent injuries and enhance coordination. Building the muscles in your abdomen, back, and hip girdle will increase your stability, balance, and speed on the field. The core muscles are also known as the powerhouse of the body. Having a strong powerhouse will help with quick, explosive movements that are needed during game time on the field. In addition, having this stability and balance in your body will protect you from injuries, even during games when muscles are overused.

Building the strength in your core is more than just crunches. Building the strength in the upper and lower core is important for balance throughout your body. Any sport that has a lot of running can affect the joints, which can lead to low-back pain. Keeping the core strong and engaged while running can reduce back pain or prevent pain altogether. Maintaining a strong core can also lead to increased speed and performance, which is enhanced by strong, stable muscles in the powerhouse. Maintaining a strong powerhouse allows your body to move more fluidly, leading to using less energy to increase time and quickness.

Keeping your core flexible is just as important as keeping the rest of the body flexible. Backbends are great poses to incorporate into your practice. After building the heat from your core work, pick any backbend pose to stretch out your front side. Slouching or rounding forward of the spine is common in runners, cyclists, golfers, and other athletes, because the movements in these sports tend to encourage a more forward posture. Core strengthening and backbends will realign and improve posture and can help prevent back pain in these athletes and others like them.

Backbends stretch more than your core. They actually stretch the whole front of your body, including the shoulders, chest, abdominal muscles, psoas, hip flexors, and quadriceps. At the same time as you stretch, you strengthen your back muscles for more support around the spine and a better balance of strength in your torso. Maintaining a safe backbend practice is largely about engaging your core. To protect your back, you should not crunch down into your low back; instead, maintain a long spine in backbends.

Spinal twisting keeps the spinal muscles mobile and your digestive system cleansed. While in a spinal twist, you are compressing and squeezing the organs, which then causes stress and a lack of circulation. When you release out of your spinal twist a rush of blood flow floods through your organs, supplying them with oxygen and nutrients. The fresh blood flow cleanses the cells of any built-up waste and helps move the impurities through your digestive tract.

KIM HARRSCH
Tennis Player

Yoga has helped me tremendously in my tennis game, not only for the obvious reasons of stretching the muscles, keeping me more flexible, and having a stronger core, but for giving me much better balance and stability. Another big thing yoga has taught me is breathing. Yoga and meditation have taught me to control my breathing, which in turn helps me to stay calm and more focused. I also use visualization in my game. I can now close my eyes and visualize what it is I want to do, for instance seeing myself hitting that great serve or shot; it works really well. In addition to my own tennis competitions I also coach middle and high school athletes. I have added to my coaching style all the yoga techniques and skills that Ryanne has taught me, and I teach them to these young athletes. I completely believe that without yoga and meditation I would not be able to compete at the level that I do today!

Spinal Twists

Spinal twists work the whole torso by stretching and twisting your abdominal muscles and the muscles of your sides and back. This stretching and twisting also increases the mobility and flexibility of your spine and all the muscles and connective tissue that connect to the vertebrae. Maintaining the mobility of the spine and gaining flexibility will increase quick, explosive movements in sport performance. It can also prevent back injuries and maintain stability for the whole body while on the field or court.

Supine Spinal Twist

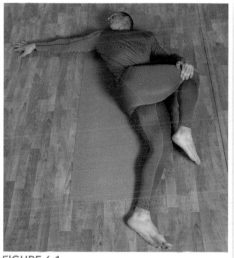

FIGURE 6.1

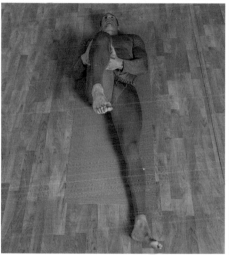

FIGURE 6.2 Supine spinal twist, modification with the knee to the chest.

Muscles

Serratus anterior, erector spinae, external and internal obliques, quadratus lumborum

1. Lie supine (on your back). Pull your right knee to your chest.
2. Straighten your left leg to the floor.
3. With your left hand, pull your right knee to the left.
4. Extend your right arm off to the right, and place your palm on the floor (figure 6.1).
5. Look to your right.
6. Hold the twist for 10 to 20 breaths, and repeat it on the other side.

Modification

Keep hugging your knee to your chest without twisting (figure 6.2).

Safety Tip

While in the twist, if you feel any discomfort in your back, lift the knee to your chest and do the modification.

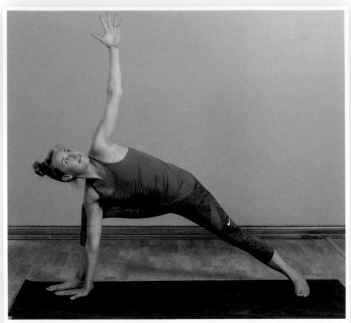

FIGURE 6.3a

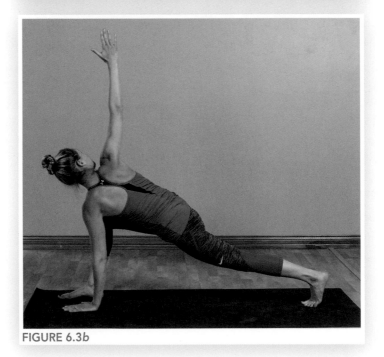

FIGURE 6.3b

Muscles

External and internal obliques, transverse abdominis, erector spinae, quadratus lumborum, gluteus maximus, adductors, psoas, pectineus, gluteus medius, tensor fasciae latae

1. From downward-facing dog pose, step your right foot forward between your hands. Turn your back heel down, and lift your torso to standing.
2. Align your right heel with your left foot arch, keeping your feet wide apart.
3. Turn your left heel back slightly past your toes so that your foot is at an angle.
4. Bend your right knee, aligning it above your right ankle.
5. Place your right palm to the floor on the inside of your right foot.
6. Have a microbend in your right elbow, helping your right knee stay above your right ankle.
7. Lean your upper back slightly back, and stack your shoulders.
8. Press down on the outer edge of your left foot, lift your arch, and your left inner thigh slightly (figure 6.3a).
9. Hold extended angle pose for 3 to 5 breaths.
10. Look down, and place your left palm on the ground.
11. Lift your left heel off the floor, balancing on the ball of your left foot.
12. Keep your spine long as you twist to the right and reach your right arm up (figure 6.3b).
13. Hold the pose for 3 to 5 breaths.
14. Look down, and come back to extended angle pose. Hold the pose for 3 to 5 breaths, and go back to twisting crescent lunge pose.
15. Do this sequence as many times as is comfortable to you, then repeat it on the other side.

Modifications

Add transitional movement between these two poses. Instead of holding the poses, start out inhaling in extended angle pose, and exhale as you transition into twisted crescent lunge pose. Follow the breath from one pose to the next pose. Instead of placing your hands on the ground, you could place them on blocks placed inside of your feet.

Safety Tip

Watch for any back discomfort when adding the twist. Maintain a long spine; do not round the spine. For major discomfort, either don't twist deeply or eliminate the twist.

Supine Spinal Twist With Knees Together

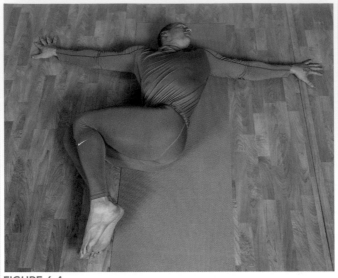

FIGURE 6.4

Muscles

Serratus anterior, erector spinae, external and internal obliques, quadratus lumborum

1. Lie on your back. Pull both knees into your chest.
2. Extend your arms out to your sides and down to the floor with the palms down.
3. Keep your knees and ankles together.
4. Lower both legs to the right (figure 6.4).
5. Tuck your left hip under your right hip to stack your hips.
6. Look to the right.
7. Hold the twist for 5 to 10 breaths, and repeat it on the other side.

Modification

Keep your knees to your chest and hug them in, lowering the legs halfway at your comfort level.

Safety Tip

If you experience discomfort in your back, keep your knees to your chest or lower your legs partway.

Supine Spinal Twist With Eagle Legs

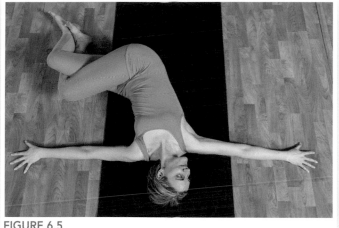

FIGURE 6.5

Muscles

Quadratus lumborum, erector spinae, external and internal obliques

1. Lie supine (on your back).
2. Reach both arms out to your sides, palms facing down.
3. Bend both knees, and plant your feet on the floor.
4. Cross your right leg over your left thigh.
5. Lift your left foot off the floor and, if possible, hook your right ankle behind your left ankle.
6. Lower both legs to your left as you look to your right (figure 6.5).
7. Hold the twist for 5 to 10 breaths, and repeat it on the other side.

Modification

If your foot cannot hook behind the opposite ankle, do not force it. Keep the feet together, and simply cross the legs.

Safety Tip

If you feel any discomfort in the knees or back, use the modification.

Seated Spinal Twist

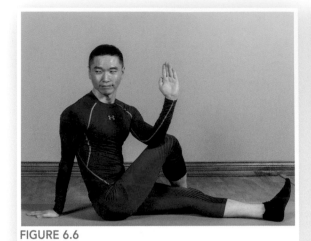

FIGURE 6.6

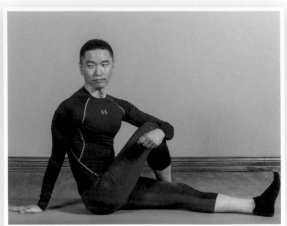

FIGURE 6.7 Seated spinal twist, modification with arm wrapped around knee.

Muscles

Quadratus lumborum, erector spinae, latissimus dorsi, external and internal obliques

1. Sit on your mat, and straighten both legs out in front of you.
2. Bend your right knee into your chest, and plant your foot on the floor outside of the left thigh.
3. Plant your right hand on the floor behind your hips.
4. Bend your left elbow, and cross your elbow to the outside of your right knee.
5. Press your right palm firmly into the floor to lengthen your spine.
6. Gently push your left elbow into your right knee to twist your torso (figure 6.6).
7. Keep the left leg long and the left foot flexed.
8. Hold the pose for 5 to 10 breaths, and repeat it on the other side.

Modification

Hug the left arm around the right knee (figure 6.7), or place a small block or blanket under the back hand to help keep a long spine.

Safety Tip

If back discomfort occurs, don't take the twist so deep. Another option is to place the right foot on the inside of the left thigh instead of crossing it to the outside of the left thigh for the spinal twist.

Twisting Chair Pose

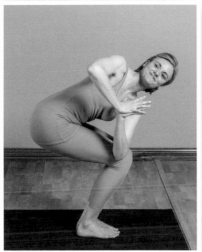

FIGURE 6.8

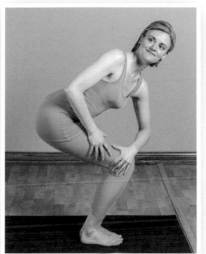

FIGURE 6.9 Twisting chair pose, modification with hands on the thigh.

Muscles

External and internal obliques, serratus anterior, erector spinae, trapezius

1. Stand at the top of your mat.
2. Bending both knees, sit your hips back.
3. Shifting your weight toward your heels, lift your chest and place your palms together.
4. Keeping your spine long, take your left elbow to the outside of your right knee.
5. Press your right palm down into the left palm, and turn your right shoulder back to take you into the twist (figure 6.8) and move your gaze up to the ceiling.
6. Keep your hips squared and your knees together.
7. Hold the pose for 5 to 10 breaths, then switch sides.

Modification

Place both hands on your right thigh, and twist to the right (figure 6.9).

Safety Tip

Maintain a long spine, and keep your hips squared so that when you go into your spinal twist you do not feel pain or discomfort in your low back.

Twisting Crescent Lunge Pose

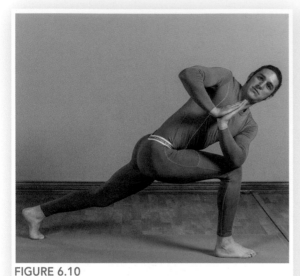

FIGURE 6.10

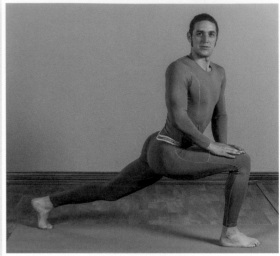

FIGURE 6.11 Twisting crescent lunge pose, modification with the hands on the thigh.

Muscles

Erector spinae, serratus anterior, trapezius

1. Start in downward-facing dog pose.
2. Step your right foot forward to the inside of your right hand.
3. Come up to standing, lifting your torso and your arms.
4. Have your feet hip-width apart.
5. Lift the left heel high.
6. Bend your right knee directly above your right ankle.
7. Place your palms in prayer position in front of your chest.
8. Take your left elbow to the outside of your right knee.
9. Press your right palm into your left palm to turn your right shoulder back for your spinal twist (figure 6.10).
10. At the same time, slowly press your left heel back and your right knee forward as you twist.
11. Hold the pose for 10 to 15 breaths, then repeat it on the other side.

Modification

Place both hands on your right thigh to twist to your right (figure 6.11).

Safety Tip

Watch for any shoulder discomfort while in this twist. If you feel any discomfort, follow the modification.

Twisting Triangle Pose

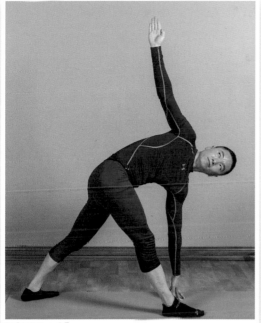

FIGURE 6.12

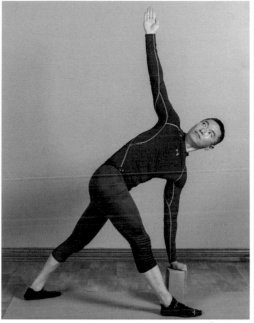

FIGURE 6.13 Twisting triangle pose, modification with a block.

Muscles

External and internal obliques, latissimus dorsi, gluteus maximus

1. From downward-facing dog pose, step your right foot forward behind your right hand.
2. Turn your back heel down.
3. Lift your torso to standing.
4. Square your hips, and straighten both legs.
5. Hinge at your hips, lengthening your spine forward.
6. Plant your left hand on the floor on the inside of your right foot.
7. Roll your right shoulder back, and reach your right arm up to the ceiling, stacking your shoulders (figure 6.12).
8. Keep your back foot planted to the floor and your hips squared.
9. Hold the pose for 10 to 20 breaths, then switch sides.

Modification

To elevate the ground, use a block on the inside of your right foot. Place your left palm on the block and your right hand on your low back, and turn your right shoulder back (figure 6.13).

Safety Tip

Avoid rounding your spine or hyperextending your knees.

Revolved Half Moon Pose

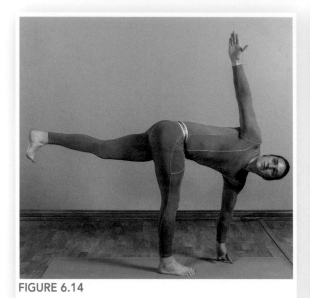

FIGURE 6.14

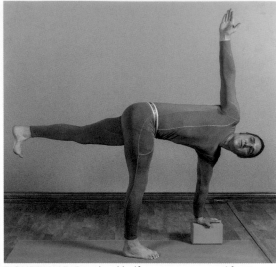

FIGURE 6.15 Revolved half moon pose, modification with a block.

Muscles

Trapezius, erector spinae, latissimus dorsi, serratus anterior, transverse abdominis, rectus abdominis

1. From downward-facing dog pose, step your right foot forward between your hands.
2. Push off your back foot to come up to balance on your right foot.
3. Plant your left hand on the ground under your left shoulder.
4. Reach your right arm to the ceiling (figure 6.14).
5. Flex your left foot, pointing your left toes to the floor, and push back through your left heel.
6. Keep your left leg at hip height and your spine long.
7. Hold the pose for 10 to 20 breaths, then switch sides.

Modifications

Place a block under your left hand to lift your torso up for a deeper spinal twist (figure 6.15). Put a bend in the standing leg if your hamstrings are tight.

Safety Tip

Avoid hyperextension by keeping a microbend in the standing knee. Don't force the twist; forcing could lead to low-back pain.

Windshield Wiper Twist

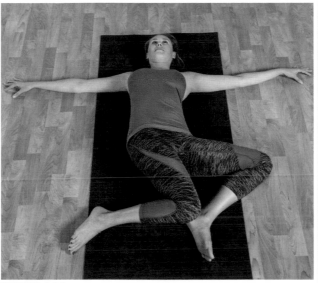

FIGURE 6.16

Muscles

Quadratus lumborum, tensor fasciae latae, external and internal obliques

1. Lie on your back on your mat.
2. Bend both knees, and plant your feet on the ground.
3. Place your left ankle on your right thigh.
4. Walk your right foot to the right edge of your mat.
5. Slowly lower both legs to the left, keeping your left ankle near your right thigh or knee.
6. Reach both arms out and away from your shoulders, and relax them to the floor.
7. Allow the weight of your left foot to bring the right knee toward the floor (figure 6.16).
8. Hold the pose for 10 to 20 breaths, then switch sides.

Modification

To intensify this stretch, slide the left heel up toward your right hip into half lotus pose, then bend the right knee and reach down with your right hand for the right foot for half hero pose.

Safety Tip

If you have knee problems, move into this pose slowly. If you feel pain, don't bend the knees so deeply; straighten the legs out more.

Cat/Cow

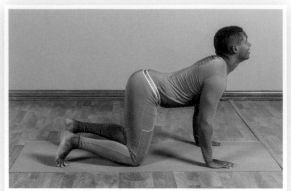

FIGURE 6.17*a*

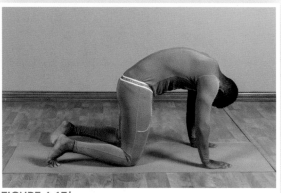

FIGURE 6.17*b*

Muscles

Rectus abdominis, erector spinae, quadratus lumborum, trapezius

1. Get on your hands and knees.
2. Inhaling, drop your belly and lift your chin and tailbone up (figure 6.17*a*).
3. Exhaling, tuck your chin to your chest. Tuck your tailbone under and press into your palms, keeping your arms straight. Round your upper back (figure 6.17*b*).
4. Repeat the movement, coordinating it with your breath for 5 to 10 rounds.

Safety Tip

If you feel any discomfort in the back, move slowly. While moving in this pose, keep the belly slightly engaged to prevent strain on the back.

Spine Rolling

Muscles

Triceps, hamstrings, gastrocnemius, soleus, quadratus lumborum, erector spinae, trapezius, rectus abdominis, pectoralis major and minor

1. Start in downward-facing dog pose (figure 6.18a).
2. Lift your heels up high, and tuck your chin to your chest.
3. Exhale completely.
4. As you inhale, tuck your tailbone under and round your spine forward (figure 6.18b) and through to an upward-facing dog pose (figure 6.18c). Lift your knees and your chin up slightly.
5. Exhaling, tuck your chin to your chest. Round your spine back to downward-facing dog pose.
6. Move with your breath between poses for 3 to 5 rounds. Move into downward facing dog or child pose for a break.

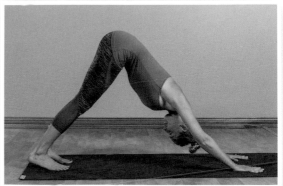

FIGURE 6.18a

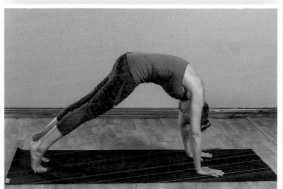

FIGURE 6.18b

Modifications

From downward-facing dog pose, shift forward to the push-up position called plank pose. Lower your hips toward the floor, pressing your hands down into the floor and lengthening your arms as you lift your chest to upward-facing dog pose. Another option is to stay in downward-facing dog pose, pressing your heels into or toward the floor.

Safety Tip

If you have any discomfort in the shoulders or low back, it would be best to do the modified version. This movement takes strength in the upper body, so it is best to be aware of the back and shoulders.

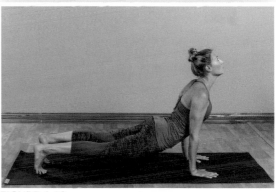

FIGURE 6.18c

Prone Spinal Twist

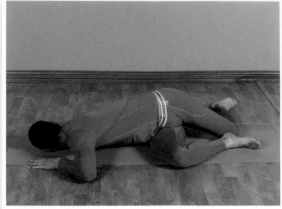

FIGURE 6.19

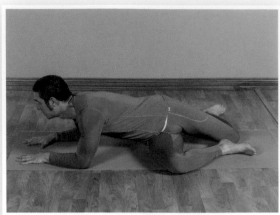

FIGURE 6.20 Prone spinal twist, modification.

Muscles

Rectus abdominis, transverse abdominis, quadratus lumborum, erector spinae, latissimus dorsi, upper trapezius

1. Sit with your knees bent and feet planted on the floor.
2. Separate your feet mat-width apart.
3. Roll both knees to the left onto your mat.
4. Circle both hands around to the front of your mat.
5. Lower to your forearms.
6. Shift your right hip under and left hip over to stack both hips.
7. Lower down to your chest as you turn your head to the right and lower your left cheek to your mat (figure 6.19).
8. Hold the twist for 10 to 15 breaths, then switch sides.

Modification

Maintain the same leg and hip positioning, but stay on your hands and keep your torso up instead of lowering your torso to the floor (figure 6.20).

Safety Tip

This pose is a deep spinal twist, so move slowly into it or follow the modification first before going deeper.

Half Lord of the Fishes Pose

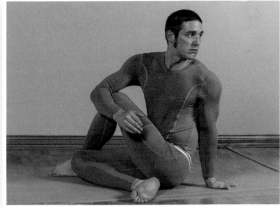

FIGURE 6.21

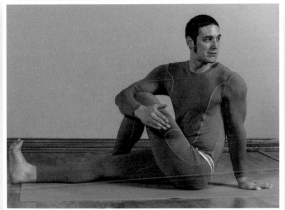

FIGURE 6.22 Half lord of the fishes pose, modification with bottom leg straight.

Muscles

External and internal obliques, trapezius, rectus abdominis

1. Sit on your mat.
2. Lengthen both legs out in front of you.
3. Bend your left knee to your chest, and plant your left foot on the floor on the outside of your right leg, keeping your left knee up by your chest.
4. Bend your right knee, and slide your right foot next to your left hip, keeping the right knee on the ground.
5. Wrap your right arm around your left knee, and hug it into your chest.
6. Plant your left hand on the floor behind your hips.
7. Press your left hand firmly down into the floor, and lengthen your spine.
8. With your right arm, hug your left knee into your chest and twist to your left (figure 6.21).
9. Hold the twist for 10 to 15 breaths, then switch sides.

Modification

Keep your right leg straight instead of bending the leg (figure 6.22). This will make the twist easier to get into if your hips and hamstrings are tight.

Safety Tip

Take your time getting into the twist to be aware of any back discomfort.

Core

The core is an important part of the body for all sports and workouts. A strong core protects the body from injuries and enhances a quality performance. Taking the time once or twice a week to focus on the core will benefit an athlete. Keep the core strong and engaged while working each core pose. For the best results take your time, stay focused on the core, and avoid any pain or discomfort.

Boat Pose

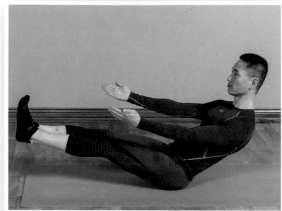

FIGURE 6.23

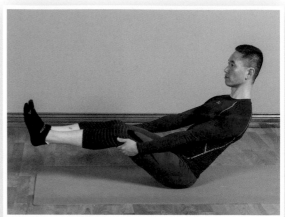

FIGURE 6.24 Boat pose, modification with bent knees.

Muscles

External and internal obliques, rectus abdominis, transverse abdominis, erector spinae

1. Sit on your mat.
2. Bend your knees, and plant your feet on the floor.
3. Sit up tall and reach your arms forward in front of you.
4. Lean your torso back so that you can balance between your sitting bones and your tailbone.
5. Straighten your legs up to a 45-degree angle (figure 6.23).
6. Keep your legs together and slightly internally rotating.
7. Keep your shoulders down and your chest lifting.
8. Hold for 5 to 10 breaths for 2 to 5 rounds.

Modification

Wrap your hands around your hamstrings, keeping your arms straight, and bend your knees, lifting your feet slightly off the floor (figure 6.24). Maintain your long spine and sitting position (between your sitting bones and tailbone).

Safety Tip

Low-back pain can be an issue in this pose, so focus on engaging your core to protect the low back.

Eagle Crunch

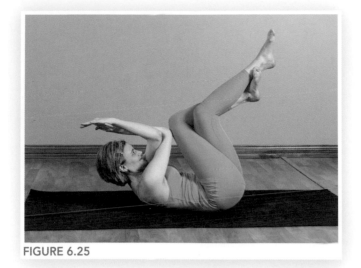

FIGURE 6.25

Muscles

Transverse abdominis, rectus abdominis

1. Lie on your back with your knees bent and feet planted on the floor.
2. Reach both arms up to the ceiling.
3. Wrap your right arm under your left elbow, and bend both elbows.
4. Wrap your hands around so that your palms meet.
5. Cross your right leg all the way over your left thigh.
6. Lift your left foot off the floor.
7. Wrap your right foot behind your left ankle, if possible.
8. When you inhale, reach your fingertips overhead and your toe tips out toward your mat.
9. As you exhale, lift your head and pull your right elbow and right thigh together (figure 6.25).
10. Keeping your head off the floor, repeat this movement, coordinating it with your breath for 2 to 4 rounds, then switch sides.

Modifications

The hands and ankles do not have to wrap all the way around. If this position is not comfortable, place your hands behind your head and do simple crunches.

Safety Tip

If you feel any discomfort in your neck and shoulders use the modification.

Knee to Elbow

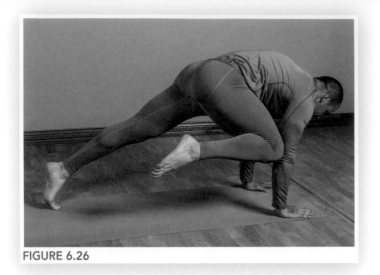

FIGURE 6.26

Muscles

Rectus abdominis, transverse abdominis

1. From downward-facing dog pose, inhale and lift your right leg up to the ceiling to a three-legged downward facing dog.
2. Exhale and shift your shoulders forward over your wrists to a plank position, bending your right knee to your elbow (figure 6.26).
3. Inhaling, lengthen your right leg back to a three-legged plank pose.
4. Exhale right knee to left elbow in plank pose.
5. Repeat this movement, coordinating with your breath for 3 sets of 10 reps each side, and switch sides.

Modification

Lower the left knee to the floor, placing it behind your hip but not directly under your hip. Just move the right knee to elbow and only extend the leg back behind you. Stick to this movement until you feel strong enough to move through this in downward-facing dog and plank movement.

Safety Tip

Cushion the knee that is down in the modification.

Lower Core Hip Lift

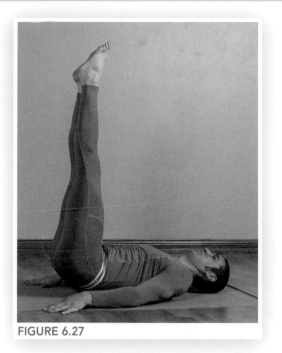

FIGURE 6.27

Muscles

Transverse abdominis

1. Lie on your back.
2. Extend both arms down your sides with your palms to the floor.
3. Lengthen both legs straight up to the ceiling.
4. Keep your shoulders down and away from your ears.
5. Exhale as you lift your hips a few inches and your toes reach for the ceiling (figure 6.27).
6. Inhale as you lower your hips slowly.
7. Repeat the sequence, coordinating it with your breath. Do two sets of 10 reps.

Modification

Bend your knees.

Safety Tip

Keep your low back on the floor to stay engaged in your core and avoid back discomfort.

Windshield Wipers

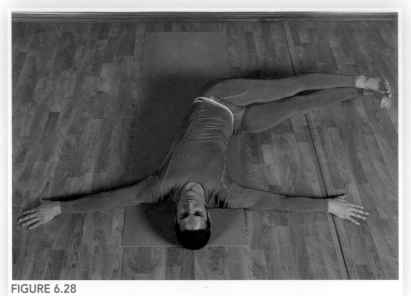

FIGURE 6.28

Muscles

External and internal obliques, rectus abdominis, transverse abdominis

1. Lie on your back
2. Extend your arms out wide at shoulder height, and place your palms facedown on the ground.
3. Straighten both legs up to the ceiling.
4. Inhale with your legs at center.
5. Exhaling, lower your legs to the right until they hover just off the floor (figure 6.28).
6. Inhaling, slowly bring your legs back up to center.
7. Exhaling, lower your legs to the left.
8. Repeat this sequence, coordinating the movements with your breath for 5 times each sides for 2 to 4 rounds.

Modification

Bend the knees to 90 degrees over the hips and move the same way with the knees bent.

Safety Tip

Keep your low back pressing into the floor while keeping your core engaged to avoid back discomfort.

Two-Leg Lower and Lift

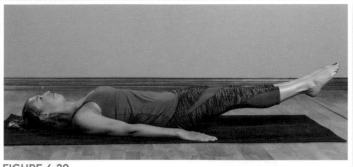

FIGURE 6.29

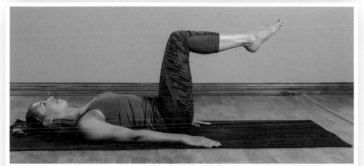

FIGURE 6.30 Two-leg lower and lift, modification with knees bent.

Muscles

Transverse abdominis

1. Lie on your mat on your back.
2. Lengthen both legs out, and reach both arms down along your sides with your palms facing down.
3. Keep your shoulders pressing down to the floor and a slight lift of your chin as you lift both legs a few inches above the mat (figure 6.29).
4. Squeeze your legs together.
5. Exhaling, lift your hips off the ground another inch or two.
6. Inhaling, slowly lower your hips to the ground.
7. Repeat this sequence as many times as you would like while keeping your core engaged.

Modification

Bend both knees to 90 degrees over the hips, lifting the knees straight up and lowering the hips slowly back down with the breath, and do the same movement, coordinating it with the breath (figure 6.30).

Safety Tip

Keep your cervical spine off the floor by slightly lifting your chin. To prevent back pain, keep your core engaged and move slowly.

One-Leg Fingertip Crunch

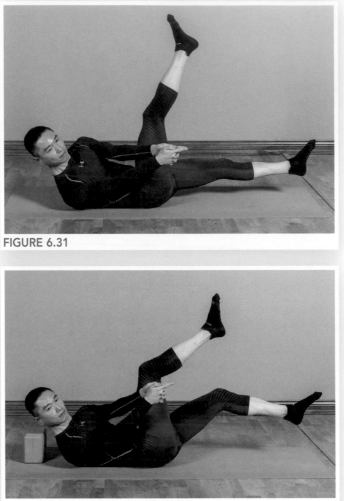

FIGURE 6.31

FIGURE 6.32 One-leg fingertip crunch, modification with leg bent.

Muscles

Rectus abdominis

1. Lie on your back.
2. Inhaling, lift both legs to the ceiling. Press your low back down into the ground.
3. Exhaling, lift your head and shoulders off the floor, and lower your left leg to a hover above the floor.
4. Reach your arms forward, and touch your fingertips behind your right hamstrings (figure 6.31).
5. Keep the head and shoulders lifted.
6. Inhaling, switch legs. Exhaling, touch your fingertips behind your left hamstrings.
7. Keep repeating the movement with the breath for as many times as you like while maintaining proper form.

Modifications

Bend the lifted leg to a 90-degree angle and, instead of touching your fingertips, reach your arms forward and focus on engaging your core through the movement (figure 6.32). If this exercise strains your neck, place a yoga block under your head and rest your head on the block like a pillow.

Safety Tip

Keep your core engaged and strong to prevent any back discomfort. Use a yoga block under your head to relax the neck in this movement.

Sliding Knee Tuck

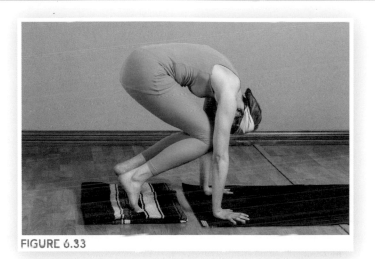

FIGURE 6.33

Muscles

Transverse abdominis

1. Use a blanket under your feet or wear socks.
2. Come to a plank pose with your hands on your mat and your feet on a noncarpeted floor. Do not have your feet on your mat.
3. Keep your shoulders away from your ears and your hands pressing into the floor.
4. Draw your belly in as you inhale.
5. Exhale as you pull both knees into your chest, sliding the feet on the floor (figure 6.33). Bring your chin to your chest.
6. Inhaling, slide your feet back to a plank pose.
7. Repeat the sequence, coordinating movement with your breath, as many times as you like.

Modification

If pulling your knees to your chest is difficult, work on holding a plank pose and pulling your belly in for your core work.

Safety Tip

While in plank pose, either holding the pose or in motion, do not sink your belly down and relax your core. Keep the body long and your core engaged to prevent any back discomfort.

Plank Pose With Heel Movement

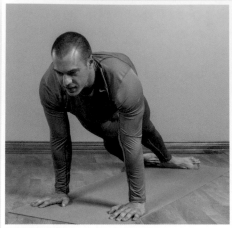

FIGURE 6.34*a*

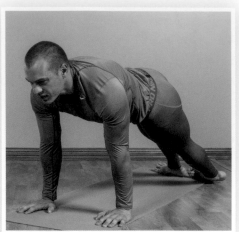

FIGURE 6.34*b*

Muscles

Transverse abdominis, external and internal obliques

1. Come to a plank pose with your feet hip-width apart.
2. Press the hands into the mat, and keep the shoulders back and away from the ears and stable above your wrists.
3. Draw your belly in tightly as you inhale.
4. Exhaling, roll both heels to the floor to your right (figure 6.34*a*) without moving your upper body.
5. Inhaling, lift your heels back up to center. Exhaling, roll your heels to the floor on your left (figure 6.34*b*).
6. Repeat the movement as many times as you like while maintaining proper form.

Modification

Hold plank pose instead of moving the heels side to side.

Safety Tip

Keep your core engaged while in the movement or holding plank pose to minimize discomfort in the back.

Bicycle

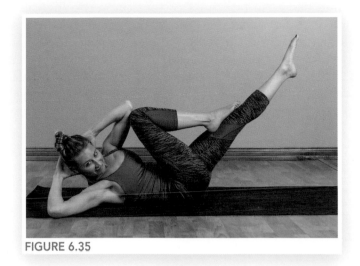

FIGURE 6.35

Muscles

Rectus abdominis, transverse abdominis

1. Lie on your back on your mat.
2. Gently place your fingers behind your head with your elbows wide.
3. Pull both knees up to your chest as you lift your head and shoulders off the floor.
4. Inhale. As you exhale, straighten your left leg out to a hover over the floor as you turn to your right and take your left elbow to your right knee and squeeze (figure 6.35).
5. Inhale, and switch sides, exhaling as you straighten the right leg and turn to your left. Repeat the sequence, following movement with your breath, while maintaining proper form for 10 to 20 reps for 3 rounds.

Modification

Instead of placing your fingers behind your head, extend your arms forward in front of you and keep the same movement of your legs with your breath.

Safety Tip

If it's easy for you to crank your head forward while your hands are behind your head, causing pain in your neck, use the modification to keep your focus on your core.

Backbends

A flexible spine can ease tightness or tension in the low back and give an athlete the mobility needed for many sports. Backbends also stretch other muscles throughout the body at the same time. Make sure to warm up before doing backbends to prevent any potential injury. I always recommend a simple spinal twist as a counterpose to backbends to protect the spine and ease tight muscles. Other counterposes to add at the end of your backbend series are downward facing dog or child's pose to relax the back.

Bridge Pose

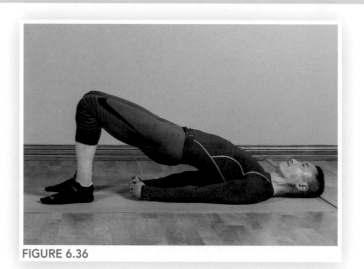

FIGURE 6.36

Muscles

Rectus abdominis, quadriceps, psoas, pectoralis major and minor, anterior deltoids, biceps, coracobrachialis

1. Lie on your back. Bend both knees, and plant your feet on the floor.
2. Lengthen both arms to the floor along your sides.
3. Press your shoulders into the mat and away from your ears.
4. Press your feet into the floor, and lift your hips.
5. Push your knees forward and your chest toward your chin to lengthen your spine.
6. Roll both shoulders under you, and walk your hands together.
7. Interlace your fingers, and press your forearms down to the mat (figure 6.36).
8. Relax your gluteal muscles, and keep lengthening your spine.

Modification

Place a block under your hips, and relax your arms to your sides.

Safety Tip

Make sure to lengthen your spine long to prevent pain in your low back.

Wheel Pose

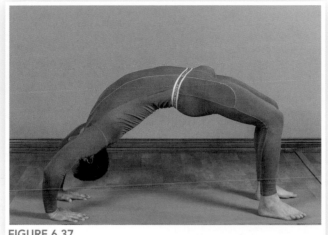

FIGURE 6.37

Muscles

Psoas, pectineus, adductor longus and brevis, sartorius, rectus femoris, rectus abdominis, transverse abdominis, deltoids, latissimus dorsi, pectoralis major, biceps, anterior neck muscles

1. Start in bridge pose (see previous description and figure 6.36). Release your hands, and place your palms under your shoulders, elbows bent.
2. Your fingertips will be pointing to your feet.
3. Keep your elbows in and parallel to each other.
4. Press your palms into your mat to lift your shoulders. Lift to the top of your head, resting softly on your head.
5. Next, press more firmly into the mat and lift all the way up, straightening your arms (figure 6.37).
6. To release, bend your elbows, tuck your chin to your chest, and lower to your shoulders first, returning to bridge pose.
7. Lower down to your back.

Modifications

Use a strap around your upper arms. This modification will allow you to use your muscles to lift up and keep you out of the joints. If this pose is too deep of a backbend or your shoulders are too tight, then bridge pose is the best modification.

Safety Tip

Shoulders and low back are areas to be cautious of in this pose. If you have really tight shoulders, work with just bridge pose. If you have a tight low back you will want to ease into this pose with bridge pose or bridge pose with a block.

Bow Pose

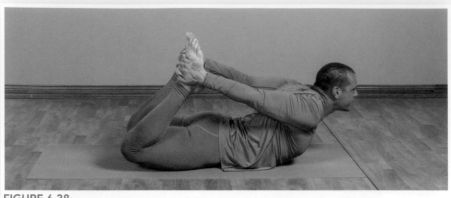

FIGURE 6.38

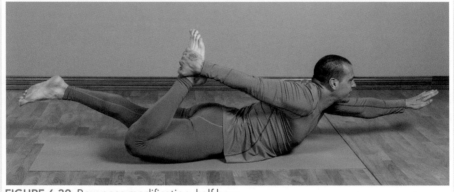

FIGURE 6.39 Bow pose modification, half bow.

Muscles

Pectoralis major, anterior deltoids, biceps, rectus abdominis, psoas, pectineus, adductor longus and brevis, sartorius, rectus femoris

1. Lie on your belly with your arms down along your sides and forehead to the floor.
2. Bend both knees.
3. Reach back and grab either your ankles or feet.
4. Press your feet back into both hands, and lift your head to look forward.
5. Lift your feet up as you keep pressing back into the hands (figure 6.38).
6. Maintain a long spine by tucking your tailbone slightly and pushing your chest forward.
7. Hold for 5 to 10 breaths for 2 to 3 rounds.

Modification

Instead of reaching back for both feet, do one side at a time (figure 6.39). Keep the opposite arm and leg lengthened down on the ground.

Safety Tip

Keep a long spine while in this pose to prevent low-back pain.

Camel Pose

Muscles

Psoas, quadriceps, pectoralis minor, biceps, rectus abdominis, anterior deltoid, psoas, anterior neck muscles, serratus anterior

1. At the top of your mat, come to an upright kneeling position.
2. Have the knees about hip-width apart.
3. Keep your tailbone lengthening downward between your knees and your gluteal muscles relaxed.
4. Lift your chest up to the ceiling, and start to push your thighs forward.
5. Tuck your chin to your chest.
6. Slowly lean back with your upper back, and place your right hand to your right heel and then your left hand to your left heel (figure 6.40).
7. If it doesn't bother your neck, relax your head back, stretching your throat.
8. Keep lifting your chest up, pushing your thighs forward and lengthening your tailbone downward.
9. Hold for 5 to 10 breaths for 2 to 3 rounds, going into child's pose as a break between each round.

Modification

Instead of reaching back with both hands, do half camel pose with one hand at a time (figure 6.41). The arm that is not reaching back for the foot reaches up to the ceiling.

Safety Tip

Knee tension may occur; cushion the knees with a blanket.

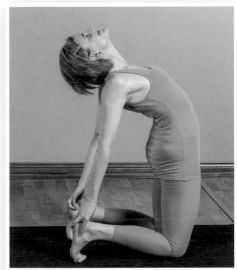

FIGURE 6.40

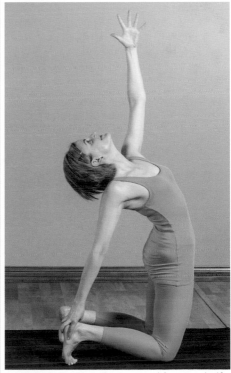

FIGURE 6.41 Camel pose modification, half camel pose.

Dancer Pose

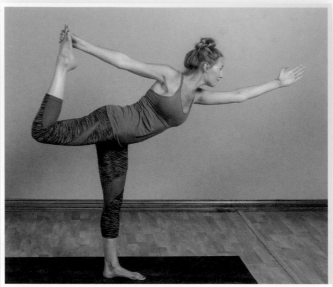

FIGURE 6.42

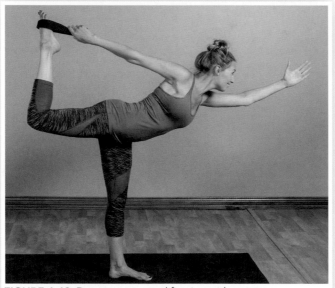

FIGURE 6.43 Dancer pose, modification with a strap.

Muscles

Psoas, pectineus, sartorius, quadriceps, hamstrings, latissimus dorsi, teres major, pectoralis minor, posterior deltoid, rectus abdominis, biceps

1. Stand tall, and put your weight on your left foot.
2. Bend your right knee, and wrap your right hand around the inside of your right foot or ankle.
3. Straighten your left arm forward in front of you.

4. Push your right foot back behind you and up into your right hand (figure 6.42).
5. Lean your torso forward as you push your foot into your hand, gazing forward.
6. Keep your tailbone tucking under and your chest lengthening forward.
7. Hold for 5 to 10 breaths.
8. Return to standing, and repeat the pose on the other side.

Modification

Loop a strap around your right foot (figure 6.43) to give you space in your back, shoulder, and knee.

Safety Tip

Maintain a long spine to avoid creating pain in your back.

Sphinx Pose

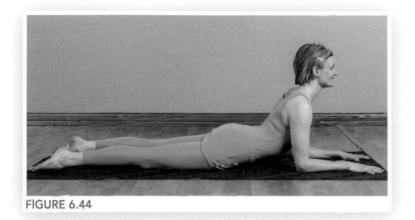

FIGURE 6.44

Muscles

Rectus abdominis, pectoralis minor

1. Lie on your belly on your mat.
2. Lift up to your forearms, aligning your shoulders over your elbows, fingers pointing forward.
3. Keep the tops of your feet pressing into the mat and your tailbone lengthening toward your heels as you press your forearms down into the mat. Energetically pull your elbows back and push your chest forward (figure 6.44).
4. Keep your shoulders down and away from your ears, and keep your gaze forward.
5. Hold the pose for 5 to 10 breaths, and relax your chest down.

Modification

Perform cobra pose (described next; see figure 6.45) instead.

Safety Tip

Keep a slight engagement of your core to protect your low back.

Cobra Pose

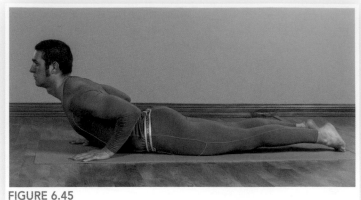

FIGURE 6.45

Muscles

Rectus abdominis, quadriceps, sartorius, pectoralis major, deltoids

1. Lie on your belly with your legs extended back, your arms down along your sides, and your forehead resting on the floor.
2. Bend your elbows, and plant your hands on the ground next to your rib cage.
3. Lift your forehead off the floor, and lengthen your chest and spine forward and upward as you press your palms down softly into the mat (figure 6.45).
4. At the same time, lengthen your legs long as you engage your quadriceps and press your feet down into the floor.
5. Keep your core engaged and your tailbone lengthening toward your heels while in this pose.

Modification

Lift your feet off the floor, lengthening through the legs as you pull your chest forward.

Safety Tip

Keep your tailbone reaching toward your heels and your core engaged to protect your low back.

Locust Pose

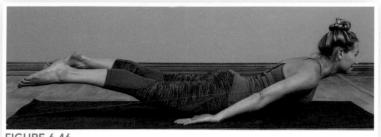

FIGURE 6.46

Muscles

Rectus abdominis, sartorius, quadriceps, deltoid, pectoralis major and minor

1. Lie on your belly with both legs extended back, your arms down along your sides, and your forehead resting on the floor.
2. Lift your forehead, and lengthen your chest forward and upward as you keep your arms along your sides, with the backs of your hands pressed against the floor.
3. At the same time, lengthen back through the balls of your feet and lift your thighs off the floor (figure 6.46).
4. Keep your core engaged and your tailbone lengthening.
5. Hold for 5 to 10 breaths

Safety Tip

Stay strong in your core, and keep your body long to prevent sinking in your low back and causing pain.

Upward-Facing Dog Pose

Muscles

Transverse abdominis, rectus abdominis, quadriceps, sartorius, iliopsoas, biceps

1. Lie on your belly with your legs long behind you and your forehead on the floor.
2. Place your palms on the floor under your shoulders, and slide your shoulders down away from your ears.
3. Press into your palms, and pull your chest forward and upward as you straighten your arms and roll your shoulders back (figure 6.47).

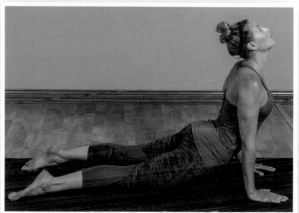

FIGURE 6.47

(continued)

4. At the same time, press into the tops of your feet and lift your knees as you engage your quadriceps and lift your thighs off the floor.

Modification

Perform cobra pose instead.

Safety tip

Use the modification if you feel back discomfort.

Wild Thing Pose

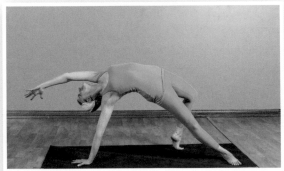

FIGURE 6.48

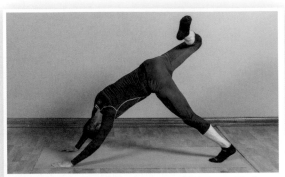

FIGURE 6.49 Wild thing pose, modification with the leg up.

Muscles

Rectus abdominis, pectoralis major, iliopsoas, quadriceps, triceps

1. Start in downward-facing dog pose. Sweep your left leg up high to the ceiling, and bend your knee to externally rotate your hip.
2. Turn to the outer edge of your right foot, keeping the right foot flexed.
3. Slowly lower the ball of the left foot to the floor on your mat behind you as you reach your left arm overhead, turning your palm to face down.
4. Press into the ball of the left foot and into your right palm as you lift your hips and chest high to the ceiling, relaxing your head back (figure 6.48). Hold for 5 to 10 breaths, and then switch sides.

Modification

From downward-facing dog pose, sweep your right leg up to the ceiling and bend the right knee to externally rotate the hip (figure 6.49). Hold this pose while breathing deeply.

Summary

The spine and core are important for the stability of the human body. When immobile and weak, these parts of the body will cause pain, tightness, or injury. Focusing on the powerhouse to build strength and mobility will increase speed, balance, and overall performance for any sport. These benefits will allow for more efficient use of energy and therefore faster times, quickness, and injury prevention.

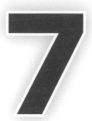

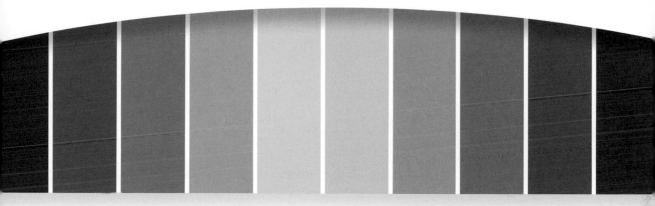

BUILDING POWER AT THE TOP: SHOULDERS, ARMS, AND NECK

Most people carry life's stresses in the neck, shoulders, and upper back. Workouts and training can also increase tightness and stiffness in the neck and shoulders. This combination can limit range of motion or cause tension headaches. The stretches in this chapter will help make your neck muscles stronger and more flexible.

When healthy and open, the shoulders can have the widest range of motion than any other area of the body. The shoulders are made up of a number of muscles, tendons, and bones that work together to allow fluid, smooth movement and wide range of motion. Proper stretching and strengthening create a strong shoulder and decrease the chance of injury. In addition, a strong, flexible shoulder can improve performance in all sports and activities. If movement of the shoulders is restricted or the shoulders lack mobility, it can lead to injuries or ongoing pain. You can work through shoulder tightness by holding simple stretches.

Many shoulder stretches also stretch down into the arms and sometimes into the hands. Lengthening and stretching the biceps, triceps, flexors, and extensors in the arms provides athletes with an advantage in many sports. In addition, these stretches prevent tendon tears and even help in the elbow joint by allowing the arm to have full extension. When the arm has the ability to extend fully without tightness, an athlete can reach out longer or up higher for that complete extension on a block, catch, pitch, or shot.

ANDY MULMUMBA
NFL Linebacker

Ryanne introduced me to visualization as we were kicking off the season. It's a known subject to me, but I have never had the chance to fully practice it until this past year. Most times I would use my relaxation time to visualize, but I have also done it before going to bed with Zen music in the background. It has helped me stay positive throughout the season, keep my confidence going, and set some goals for myself that I would be looking to accomplish in the near future. I turned my escape from the real world into visualization, because nothing can fail if you have a positive mindset within every aspect of your life. I can surely attest to the positive effects visualization can have on people when it's done correctly and consistently. Mixing my yoga practice and visualization has helped me control my mind, eliminate the unnecessary thoughts, but most of all I stayed positive and confident in my abilities as a football player, and it made me a better person.

Shoulders and Arms

Keeping the shoulders and arms loose and mobile not only decreases tension from daily life stressors but increases range of motion for sports. Take the time to hold the poses that provide the best stretch for you, and incorporate new ones to stay balanced in your mobility.

Eagle Arms

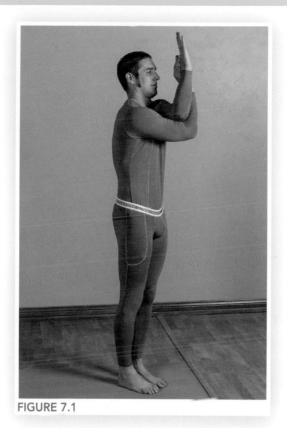

FIGURE 7.1

Muscles

Rhomboids, middle trapezius, deltoids, supraspinatus, infraspinatus, teres minor, teres major

1. Standing at the top of your mat, extend your arms out in front of you, palms facing each other.
2. Hook your right elbow under your left elbow, and bend both elbows.
3. Wrap your right forearm around your left forearm, and bring your palms together.
4. Push your forearms forward and away from your chest, and lift your fingers toward the ceiling (figure 7.1).
5. Hold the stretch for 5 to 15 breaths, then switch sides.

Modification

If your palms do not touch, touch the backs of your hands together and focus on the elbows staying bent and forearms pushing forward and up.

Safety Tip

As you push your forearms forward, move slowly to avoid overstretching.

Puppy Pose Variation

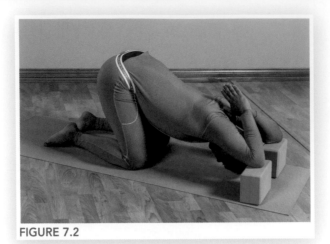

FIGURE 7.2

Muscles

Triceps, trapezius, serratus anterior, teres major, subscapularis

1. Place two blocks at the top of your mat.
2. Come to your hands and knees in front of your blocks.
3. Place your right elbow on top and at the front edge of the block to your right.
4. Place your left elbow on top and to the front edge of the block to your left.
5. Bring your palms together.
6. Relax your head down toward the floor.
7. Bend both elbows, and have your thumbs touch your upper back (figure 7.2).
8. Shift your hips back slowly to deepen this stretch.

Modification

Do not bend the elbows. With really tight shoulders, bending the elbows is too much of a challenge.

Safety Tip

As you lower your head to or toward the floor, go slowly as you go deeper into this pose.

Wall Stretch

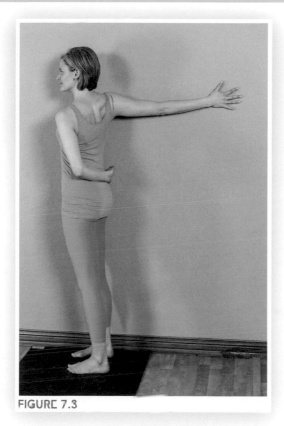

FIGURE 7.3

Muscles

Pectoralis minor, deltoids, biceps, teres major, subscapularis, serratus anterior, flexor muscles of the forearm

1. Stand up close to a wall, facing the wall.
2. Extend your right arm off to the right, placing your palm on the wall at three o'clock.
3. Turn your whole body to the left, leaning your right armpit toward the wall.
4. Wrap your left arm behind your back (figure 7.3).
5. Keep turning your left shoulder to the left to deepen this stretch.
6. Repeat with the same arm at two and one o'clock, then switch arms.

Modification

If you have very tight shoulders, turn only halfway to the left.

Safety Tip

Take this stretch slowly, making sure not to overstretch, especially if your shoulders tend to be tight.

Simple Twist With Shoulder Stretch

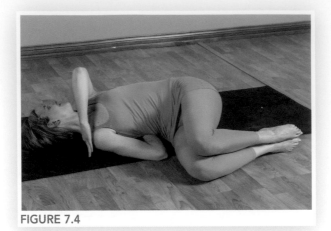

FIGURE 7.4

Muscles

Anterior deltoid

1. Lie on your back with both arms extended out wide and palms facing down.
2. Bend your knees, and plant your feet on the floor with the feet together.
3. Lift your right hip off the floor.
4. Bend your right elbow, and slide your hand under your back only wrist deep.
5. Slide the hand up toward your right shoulder blade and touch your right shoulder with your left hand.
6. Relax your right hip back to the ground.
7. Relax both knees to the floor on your right (figure 7.4).
8. Look to your left.
9. Hold for 10 to 20 breaths.
10. Switch sides.

Modification

Keep the knees up instead of lowering them to the side.

Safety Tip

This twist can require a deep bend in the elbow, so be mindful not to cause discomfort or pain in the elbow. If you feel any pain, come out of the pose immediately.

Thread the Needle Pose

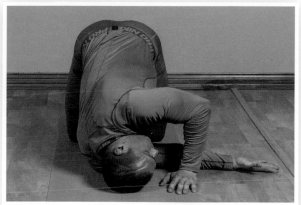

FIGURE 7.5

Muscles

Deltoids, trapezius, supraspinatus, infraspinatus

1. Start on your hands and knees, stacking your shoulders above your wrists and your hips above your knees.
2. Slide your right arm to the left between your left arm and leg.
3. Bend your left elbow to lower your right shoulder and ear to the floor, sinking onto the right shoulder (figure 7.5).
4. Press your left palm into the floor to twist your left shoulder back, stretching your right shoulder
5. Hold for 5 to 10 breaths.
6. Switch sides.

Modification

If you are not able to lower completely to the floor, place a block under your head.

Safety Tip

Don't put all of your weight on your head. Sink your weight on your shoulder, not on your cervical spine.

Shoulder Rotation With Strap

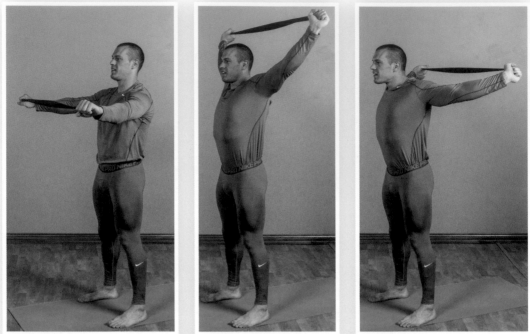

FIGURE 7.6a   FIGURE 7.6b   FIGURE 7.6c

Muscles

Pectoralis major and minor, subscapularis, teres major

1. Stand with your feet hip-width apart. Stand tall as you would in mountain pose.
2. Holding a yoga strap in both hands, extend your arms forward in front of you (figure 7.6a).
3. Slide your hands just past shoulder-width apart, keeping your arms straight and maintaining this grip.
4. As you inhale, lift your arms overhead, keeping your arms straight (figure 7.6b).
5. Exhaling, slowly allow the arms to fall back behind you (figure 7.6c).
6. Slide the hands apart along the strap until your arms go all the way through.
7. Inhale back up, and exhale forward.
8. Repeat this sequence, coordinating movement with your breath for 2 sets of 10 reps.

Modification

Instead of moving the arms all the way through behind you, have the arms go overhead until you feel the stretch, then hold it.

Safety Tip

If you have had any recent shoulder injury, do not do this movement.

Crisscross Pose

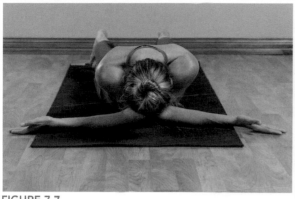

FIGURE 7.7

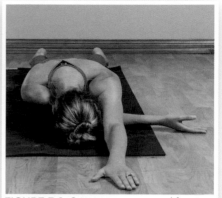

FIGURE 7.8 Crisscross pose, modification with one arm.

Muscles

Deltoids, trapezius, supraspinatus, infraspinatus, rhomboids

1. Lie on your abdomen, resting on your forearms.
2. Turn your right palm faceup.
3. Take your right hand behind your left arm and slide it to your left, staying on the right elbow.
4. Turn your left palm faceup and slide your left hand to the right, staying up on the elbow (figure 7.7).
5. If you have space, keep sliding the arms apart, staying on your elbows.
6. Relax your head down toward the floor, resting your weight on your arms.
7. To deepen this stretch, curl your toes under and push your body weight forward, then relax your head down.
8. Hold for 10 to 20 breaths, and switch arms.

Modification

Move your right arm across to the left. Instead of crossing your left arm to the left, reach your left arm out overhead and rest your head and body weight down to the floor (figure 7.8).

Safety Tip

If you have had a shoulder injury or other shoulder problems, you may want to avoid this stretch.

Open Chest Pose

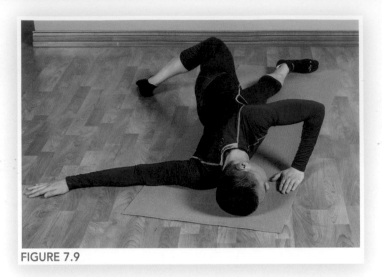

FIGURE 7.9

Muscles

Pectoralis major, deltoid, subscapularis, teres major, flexor muscles of the forearm

1. Lie on your abdomen.
2. Reach your right arm long, out to the right at shoulder level.
3. Bend your left elbow, and plant your left palm under your left shoulder.
4. Turn your head, and look to the left.
5. Bend your left knee and flip your left foot, placing it on the ground behind your right knee. Lift your left knee to the ceiling.
6. Press your left palm into the floor to turn your left shoulder to the left (figure 7.9).
7. Hold for 10 to 20 breaths, and switch arms.

Modification

Instead of flipping your left leg behind the right, just roll to your right side.

Safety Tip

If you have had a recent shoulder injury, you should not do this pose.

Supported Fish Pose With Shoulder Stretch

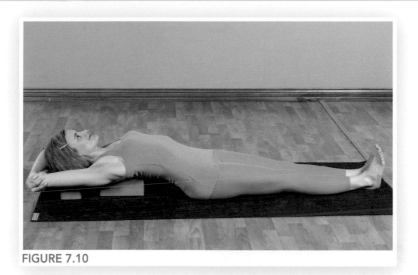

FIGURE 7.10

Muscles

Teres major, subscapularis, serratus anterior, pectoralis minor, triceps

1. Use two yoga blocks.
2. Place the first yoga block on your mat on the lowest level lengthwise with your mat.
3. Place the second yoga block sideways in front of the first yoga block.
4. Sit down in front of the first yoga block about a foot away, facing away from the blocks.
5. Lower backward onto your forearms.
6. Slowly lower back onto the first yoga block, which is positioned between your shoulder blades.
7. Relax your head back onto the second yoga block.
8. Straighten your legs forward, and draw them together.
9. Reach your arms up to the ceiling, and bend at both elbows.
10. Clasp opposite elbows.
11. Relax your forearms overhead toward the floor (figure 7.10).
12. Hold for 10 to 20 breaths.
13. Switch arms.

Modification

If your shoulders are too tight and this pose does not feel good, take your arms instead out to the sides and work the backs of your hands to the floor.

Safety Tip

The second block is like a pillow for your head. Use any level of the block that will support your head and feel good for your neck.

Wide-Legged Forward Fold With Strap

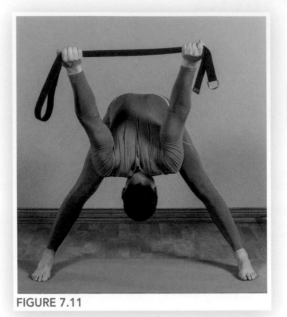

FIGURE 7.11

Muscles

Anterior deltoid, pectoralis major and minor

1. Stand on your mat with your feet wide apart, longer than one leg-width apart.
2. Hold a yoga strap behind you in both hands with your hands hip-width apart or farther.
3. Fold your torso forward and downward into a wide-legged forward fold. Lift both arms up off your back, and reach them toward the ceiling (figure 7.11).
4. Hold the legs steady, and breathe as you relax the arms into the stretch.
5. Hold for 10 to 20 breaths.

Modification

Separate the hands wide apart along the strap if your shoulders are really tight. Slowly work your hands closer together in time.

Safety Tip

Ease into this pose, especially if your shoulders are tight.

Forward Fold With Shoulder Stretch

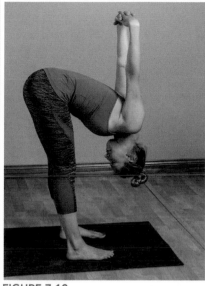

FIGURE 7.12

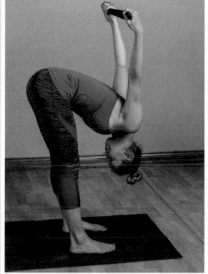

FIGURE 7.13 Forward fold with shoulder stretch, modification with strap.

Muscles

Anterior deltoid, pectoralis major and minor

1. Stand at the top of your mat with your feet about hip-width apart.
2. Reach the arms around behind you, and interlace your fingers, bringing the palms together.
3. Inhaling, lift your chest. Exhaling, fold forward. Lift your arms off your low back, bringing your knuckles toward the ceiling (figure 7.12).
4. Hold the pose for 5 to 10 breaths, then return to standing. Switch the grip in your hands by placing the opposite thumb on top, and fold forward for the second round.

Modifications

Having the palms together makes the shoulder stretch more difficult. Separate the hands, but keep the fingers interlaced to add more space for the shoulder stretch. If this modification is still difficult for the shoulders, use a yoga strap and separate the hands farther apart to ease into the shoulder stretch (figure 7.13).

Safety Tip

If your shoulders are tight, do the modification with a strap, being mindful to avoid discomfort.

Cow Face Arms

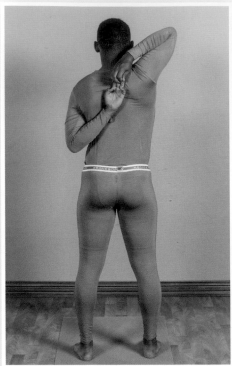

FIGURE 7.14

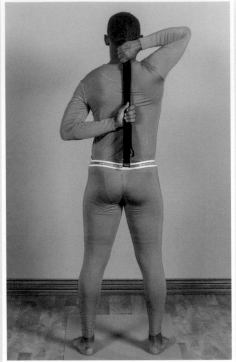

FIGURE 7.15 Cow face arms, modification with strap.

Muscles

Deltoids, infraspinatus, supraspinatus

1. Standing at the top of your mat, bend your left elbow, internally rotating the shoulder, and place the back of your left hand on your low back.
2. At the same time, reach your right arm overhead, externally rotating the shoulder, and bend your right elbow, placing your right hand on your upper back.
3. Slowly slide both hands together, and interlace your fingers (figure 7.14).
4. Keep your right elbow pointing up to the ceiling, lifting your chest up to stand tall while in this stretch.
5. Hold the position for 10 to 15 breaths, then switch sides.

Modification

If your fingers do not meet, hold a yoga strap in the top hand, then drop it down to the other hand (figure 7.15).

Safety Tip

If your shoulders are tight, follow the modification using a strap.

Half Crisscross Pose

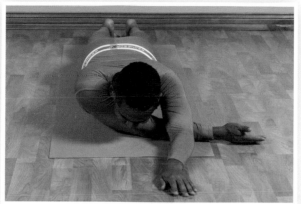

FIGURE 7.16

Muscles

Deltoids, trapezius, supraspinatus, infraspinatus, rhomboids

1. Lie on your belly, resting on your forearms.
2. Slide your forearms forward so that your elbows are just past your shoulders, not in line with them.
3. Turn your right palm faceup, and slide your right arm behind your left triceps, lowering down on your triceps and not your deltoid.
4. Slide your left arm forward, lowering your left shoulder toward the floor.
5. Relax your body weight down and drop your forehead toward (or all the way to) the floor (figure 7.16).
6. Hold the pose for 10 to 15 breaths, then switch sides.

Modification

Keep your head and chest up instead of down toward the floor. This modification will ease the intensity of the stretch.

Safety Tip

If your shoulders are tight, use the modification and gradually work your way into the full stretch.

Open Chest Pose With 90-Degree Arm

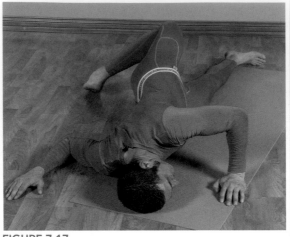

FIGURE 7.17

Muscles

Pectoralis major and minor, anterior deltoid

1. Lie on your abdomen.
2. Reach your right arm off to your right side, and bend your elbow, relaxing your arm on the floor at a 90-degree angle.
3. Align your right elbow up with your right shoulder and your right wrist with your right elbow.
4. Place your left palm under your left shoulder and look to your left, resting your head on the floor.
5. Bend your left knee as you lift your left leg, and flip your left leg behind your right leg (figure 7.17).
6. Push into the floor with your left palm to roll your left shoulder back for a deeper stretch.
7. Hold the pose for 10 breaths, and switch sides.

Modification

If this stretch is too intense, do open chest pose (figure 7.9) with the arm straight.

Safety Tip

Enter into this pose slowly.

Neck

One of the main causes of headaches is tension from tightness in the neck. The tightness can start either in the shoulders or the neck and move up to where the muscles attach at the base of the skull. Practicing simple neck stretches or movements can loosen up and calm these tense areas to decrease the chance of headaches and improve the range of motion in your neck.

Seated Half Neck Roll

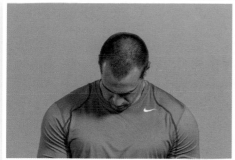
FIGURE 7.18a

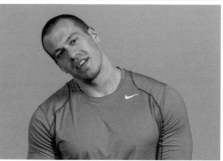
FIGURE 7.18b

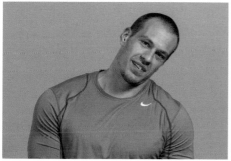
FIGURE 7.18c

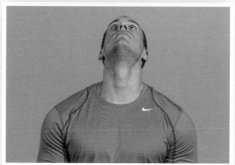
FIGURE 7.18d

Muscles

Levator scapulae, trapezius, sternocleidomastoid, scalenes

1. Sit in a comfortable position.
2. Rest your hands on your thighs.
3. Sit up tall, lengthening through the top of your head.
4. Relax your head forward, keeping your shoulders down (figure 7.18a).
5. Slowly roll your head to your right shoulder, and stop (figure 7.18b).
6. Gently roll your head forward and to your left shoulder, and stop (figure 7.18c).
7. Move gently and slowly with your breath, feeling the stretch as you move your head.
8. If you feel a stretch, hold that spot and breathe.
9. Repeat the same movement with your head tilted back (figure 7.18d).

Modification

If your neck is tight, hold each position—forward, right side, and left side—for 2 to 5 breaths each hold.

Safety Tip

If you have any past injuries to your neck, make sure to follow the modification and go easy on your neck.

Hands and Knees Neck Roll

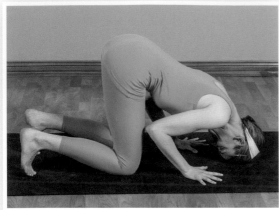

FIGURE 7.19*a*

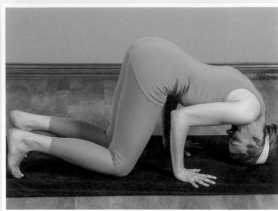

FIGURE 7.19*b*

Muscles

Levator scapulae, trapezius

1. Start on your hands and knees.
2. Bend your elbows into your rib cage as you lower your head to the mat between your hands, placing the space just above your hairline to the mat (figure 7.19a).
3. Use your hands for balance and control.
4. Slowly shift your hips forward, allowing you to roll over the top of your head, only resting but not pushing your head down (figure 7.19b).
5. Roll as far forward as is comfortable for your neck or until your chin touches your chest.
6. Slowly shift your hips back, rolling over the head and back to where you started.

Modification

Perform seated half neck roll (figure 7.18).

Safety Tip

The neck is a sensitive part of the body. Take this move slowly and gently, being mindful not to compress the cervical spine and without overstretching the muscles in your neck.

Arms

Maintaining loose shoulders and arms can prevent major muscle tears or long-term problems resulting from repetitive motion. Following just a few of these stretches can help with mobility and flexibility in the arms.

Wrist Stretch With Palms on Floor

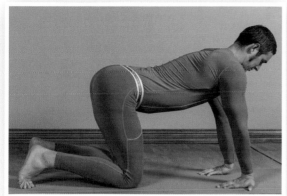

FIGURE 7.20

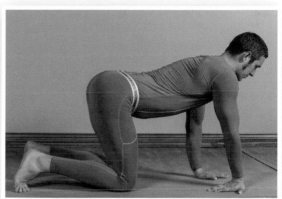

FIGURE 7.21 Wrist stretch with palm on floor, modification with one hand.

Muscles

Flexor carpi radialis, flexi carpi ulnaris, brachioradialis, flexor digitorum profundus, lumbricals

1. Begin on your hands and knees on your mat.
2. Turn your right hand clockwise so that your fingers point to your right knee.
3. Turn your left hand counterclockwise so that your fingers point to your left knee.
4. Keep both palms planted on the floor and your shoulders away from your ears.
5. Slowly shift your hips back toward your heels, and stop when you feel a stretch in your wrists and forearms (figure 7.20).
6. Hold the stretch for 5 to 10 breaths. Slowly shift your hips forward to release your hands, and sit back into child's pose.

Modification

Do one hand at a time (figure 7.21) to ease the intensity of this stretch.

Safety Tip

Move slowly to get into this stretch, and follow the modification.

Prayer Hands

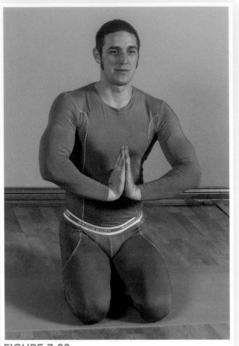

FIGURE 7.22

Muscles

Flexor carpi radialis, flexi carpi ulnaris, brachioradialis, flexor digitorum profundus, lumbricals

1. Bring both palms together in front of your chest.
2. Press your palms together as you lower your wrists and lift your elbows (figure 7.22).
3. Hold the stretch for 10 breaths, then relax. Repeat the stretch 3 times.

Modification

Instead of lowering the wrists, hold the palms together and breathe.

Safety Tip

If you feel any wrist discomfort, follow the modification.

Reverse Prayer Hands

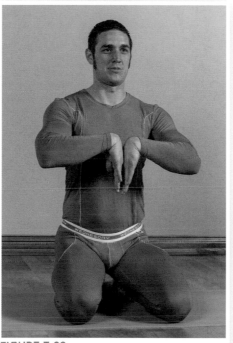

FIGURE 7.23

Muscles

Flexor carpi radialis, flexi carpi ulnaris, brachioradialis, flexor digitorum profundus, lumbricals

1. Bring the backs of your hands together with your fingers pointing down.
2. Press the backs of your hands together as you lift your wrists and lower your elbows (figure 7.23).
3. Hold the position for 10 breaths, and release. Repeat the stretch 3 times.

Modification

Hold the backs of the hands together without lifting the wrists.

Safety Tip

If you feel any wrist discomfort, follow the modification.

Summary

Staying strong and flexible in the shoulders can improve performance in all sports and activities. Shoulder mobility also increases flexibility in the arms and neck. This improves arm extension, which will help an athlete block a shot or extend for a catch. Adding these stretches to your routine will benefit your athletic training and performance.

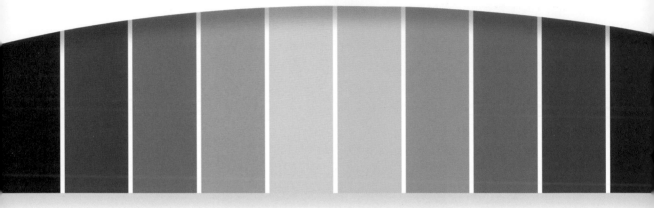

WAKING UP SMALL MUSCLES: BALANCE POSES

This chapter focuses on the ankles and feet. The poses shown in this chapter are meant to stretch and strengthen the lower part of the legs. The muscles listed for each pose are located in the lower parts of your legs, feet, and ankles. These poses are also beneficial for other areas of the body; however, the chapter focuses primarily on the benefits to the lower part of leg.

The lower part of the legs consist of many little bones, tendons, and muscles. During training athletes usually don't think they have to stretch or strengthen the feet or ankles. The thought may never have crossed your mind. People tend to only be reminded of this area when they are achy, in pain, or injured. On a daily basis, you put your feet through a lot of hard work from the moment you step out of bed in the morning to the moment you climb back in at the end of the day. With all this daily work, tight and stiff ankles and feet can become a problem. When initially taking on a yoga practice, slowing down the practice to narrow in on a precise movement and balancing on one foot or the ankles can be very difficult and even uncomfortable. It is difficult at first because the muscles in the feet are working to build strength. As you do these poses more often, you will gain not only flexibility in your lower legs, you will also gain strength. Having both strength and flexibility helps prevent major injury that could possibly put you out for the season or longer. At any moment during a game, you can misstep, roll your ankle, or get stepped on. At these moments, having a strong and flexible ankle will get you back to playing sooner than expected.

MELISSA FLUCKE

University of Minnesota–Twin Cities Track and Field

As an NCAA Division I pole vaulter and high jumper and now as a runner, practicing yoga has allowed me to put things into perspective. It has taught me how to stay in the moment while competing, as well as slow my mind and body down when I get nervous or start overthinking the process. I use the relaxation and meditation skills yoga has taught me in my everyday life, and I will continue to do so wherever my professional and athletic life takes me.

Warrior III Pose

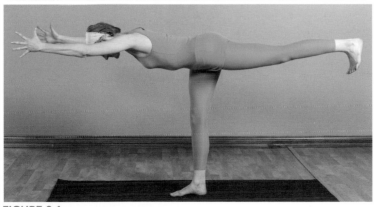

FIGURE 8.1

Muscles

Peroneus longus and brevis, gastrocnemius, tibialis anterior, extensor hallucis, adductor hallucis, extensor digitorum, flexor digitorum, soleus, adductor digiti minimi, trochlea tali, flexor hallucis, tibialis posterior

(continued)

1. Start in downward-facing dog pose. Step your right foot forward between your hands.
2. Reach both arms overhead.
3. Push off your back foot, and lift up to balance on your right foot.
4. Flex your left foot, keeping your toes pointing to the ground.
5. Straighten your left leg long, and keep your left heel in line with your left hip.
6. Square your hips.
7. Keep the torso in line with your hips and left leg.
8. Draw your navel in toward your spine.
9. Reach your arms overhead (figure 8.1).
10. Focus your gaze down to the ground.
11. Hold for 5 to 10 breaths.
12. Repeat the pose on the other leg.

Modification

Place a yoga block standing tall on the floor directly under your shoulders. Place both hands on the block before coming up to balance, then follow the same directions with your hands on the block (figure 8.2). Slowly take one hand off the block, and reach your arm out to your side. Work on the same sequence with the other arm until both hands are no longer on the block and you are balancing.

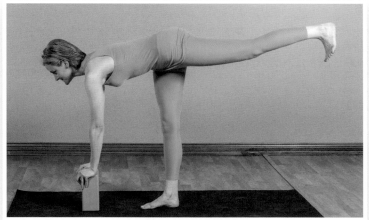

FIGURE 8.2 Warrior III, modification with block.

Safety Tip

Reaching both arms overhead can cause discomfort or pain on the shoulders, neck, or back. Allow your arms to be reaching out of your shoulders as if you were flying, or have them down along your sides reaching behind you.

Half Moon Pose

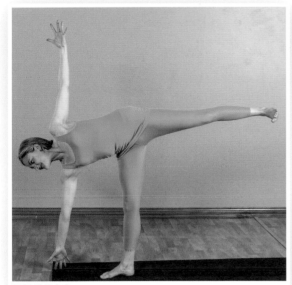

FIGURE 8.3

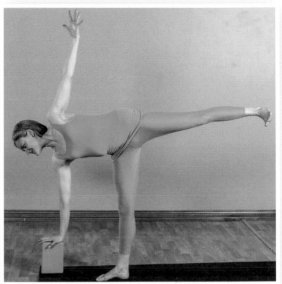

FIGURE 8.4 Half moon pose, modification with block.

Muscles

Gastrocnemius, soleus, peroneus longus and brevis, gastrocnemius, tibialis anterior, extensor hallucis, adductor hallucis, extensor digitorum, flexor digitorum, soleus, adductor digiti minimi, trochlea tali, flexor hallucis, tibialis posterior

1. Start in downward-facing dog pose. Step your right foot forward between your hands.
2. Push off your left foot to balance on your right foot.
3. Place your right palm or fingertips on the floor under your right shoulder.
4. Roll your left shoulder and hip back, opening the front of your body to the left.
5. Flex your left foot, and lift your left leg to hip height (figure 8.3).
6. Stack your shoulders and hips.
7. Keep your tailbone slightly tucked under to maintain length in the spine.
8. Hold for 5 to 10 breaths and step back to downward facing dog or run through a vinyasa.
9. Repeat the pose on the other side.

Modification

Place a block under your right hand (figure 8.4) to help with balance and any tight hamstrings that restrict you from touching the floor.

Safety Tip

Watch for hyperextension in the standing leg. Put a microbend in the knee to stay strong in the leg.

Tree Pose

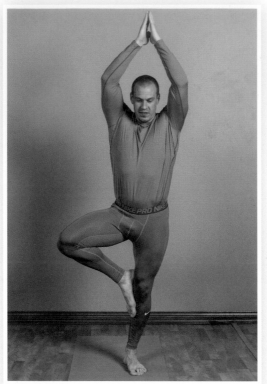

FIGURE 8.5

Muscles

Gastrocnemius, soleus, peroneus longus and brevis, tibialis anterior, extensor hallucis, adductor hallucis, extensor digitorum, flexor digitorum, adductor digiti minimi, trochlea tali, flexor hallucis, tibialis posterior

1. Standing at the top of your mat, bend your right knee to your chest, balancing on your left foot.
2. Place the bottom of your right foot on your left inner thigh.
3. Stay standing tall as you reach your arms overhead and bring your palms together in prayer (figure 8.5).
4. Hold for 5 to 10 breaths and take a forward fold between poses.
5. Repeat the pose on the other leg.

Modifications

The bottom of your right foot can be anywhere along the inside of your left leg. If your balance is off today, just place your right heel on your left ankle, leaving the ball of your right foot on the ground like a kickstand for support.

Safety Tip

Balance poses take practice, so always start with the modification first or use the yoga props and work your way to the full pose.

Standing Split

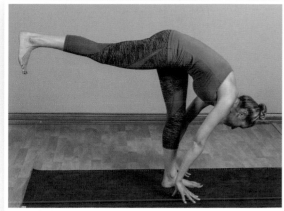

FIGURE 8.6

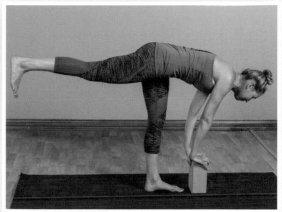

FIGURE 8.7 Standing split, modification with block.

Muscles

Gastrocnemius, soleus, peroneus longus and brevis, tibialis anterior, extensor hallucis, adductor hallucis, extensor digitorum, flexor digitorum, adductor digiti minimi, trochlea tali, flexor hallucis, tibialis posterior, Achilles tendon

1. Start in warrior III pose.
2. Take both hands down to the floor as you lift your back leg up toward the ceiling.
3. Walk your hands back to your left foot and fold forward, taking your nose to your knee or shin (figure 8.6).
4. Place the left hand around your left ankle and then the right hand around your left ankle.
5. Keep lifting your right leg up to the ceiling only as far as your body will allow you.
6. Hold for 5 to 10 breaths and step back to downward facing dog or run through a vinyasa. Repeat this pose on the other leg.

Modification

Place a block standing tall on the floor under your chest to rest both hands on (figure 8.7). Work your way to the next level of the block until your hands eventually touch the floor. In the meantime, keeping the block standing tall, wrap one hand around your calf muscle or ankle to work on your balance.

Safety Tip

Avoid hyperextension of the standing leg. Maintain a microbend of the knee to keep the knee strong and stay away from future knee problems.

Sugar Cane Pose

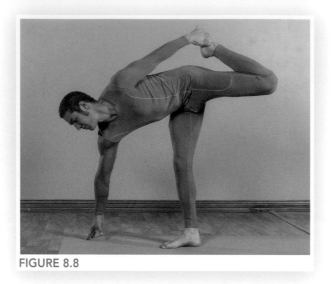

FIGURE 8.8

Muscles

Gastrocnemius, soleus, peroneus longus and brevis, tibialis anterior, extensor hallucis, adductor hallucis, extensor digitorum, flexor digitorum, adductor digiti minimi, trochlea tali, flexor hallucis, tibialis posterior

1. Start in half moon pose balancing on your right leg.
2. Bend your left knee, and with your left hand reach back and clasp your outer left foot or ankle (figure 8.8).
3. Press your foot back into your hand, opening your chest.
4. Gaze down toward the ground, slowly bringing your right hand down to the ground.
5. Hold for 5 to 10 breaths.
6. To come out of the pose, release the left foot, lengthening the left leg back to half moon pose. Then bend the right knee and slowly step back to downward facing dog or run through a vinyasa.
7. Repeat the pose on the opposite side.

Modification

Place a block under your right hand, and focus on the balance in half moon pose.

Safety Tip

This pose is also a backbend and shoulder opener, so make sure your body is warmed up in preparation for it.

Warrior III Pose to Jiva Squat

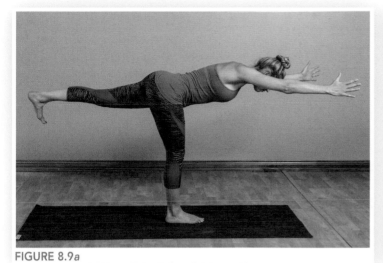

FIGURE 8.9a

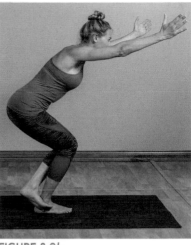

FIGURE 8.9b

Muscles

Gastrocnemius, soleus, peroneus longus and brevis, tibialis anterior, extensor hallucis, adductor hallucis, extensor digitorum, flexor digitorum, adductor digiti minimi, trochlea tali, flexor hallucis, tibialis posterior, Achilles tendon

1. Start in warrior III pose (figure 8.9a) with your right leg as the standing leg.
2. Inhale and bend your right knee, lowering to a squat.
3. As you descend, bend the left knee and wrap your left ankle around your right ankle, keeping your arms reaching overhead (figure 8.9b).
4. Exhale and slowly straighten your right leg, and lift back up to warrior III.
5. Do 5 of these movements on each leg with your breath recovery between each side in downward facing dog or forward fold, then repeat the same sequence on the left leg.

Modification

Place a yoga block standing tall on your mat directly under your chest for balance. Do the same movement with both hands on the block (figure 8.10).

Safety Tip

If you have troubled knees, it might be best to hold warrior II pose or warrior III pose to avoid discomfort, pain, or instability.

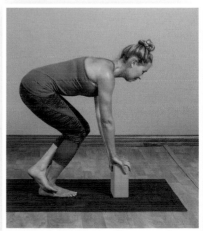

FIGURE 8.10 Warrior III pose to jiva squat, modification with a block.

Warrior III Pose With Leg Movement

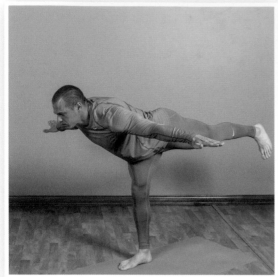

FIGURE 8.11a

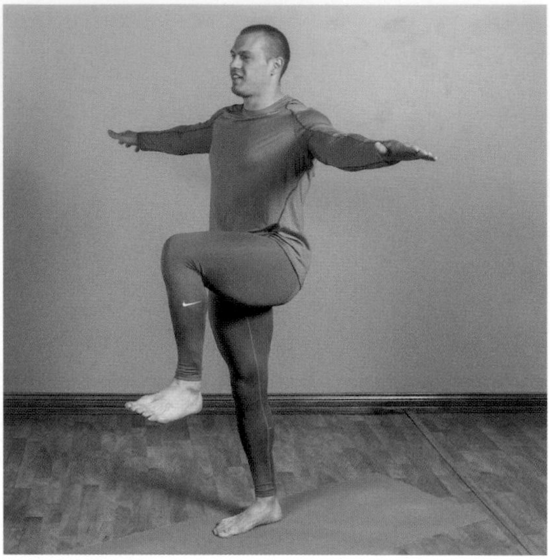

FIGURE 8.11b

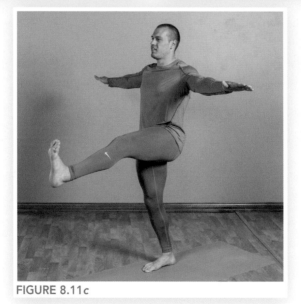

FIGURE 8.11c

Muscles

Gastrocnemius, soleus, peroneus longus and brevis, tibialis anterior, extensor hallucis, adductor hallucis, extensor digitorum, flexor digitorum, adductor digiti minimi, trochlea tali, flexor hallucis, tibialis posterior

1. Start in warrior III pose (figure 8.11a).
2. Inhale and bend your left knee to your chest, and lift your torso up to standing on your right leg with the left knee to your chest and arms overhead or out to the sides (figure 8.11b).

3. Flex your left foot, exhale, and straighten your left leg out in front of you, keeping your arms straight over your head or out to the sides (figure 8.11c).

4. Keeping your left leg straight, inhale, and slowly circle your left leg to the left and behind you, back into warrior III pose on the exhale.

5. Follow this movement sequence five times, and repeat it on the other side.

Modification

Have a yoga block on your mat under your chest while in warrior III pose. Keep it there during this sequence for any moment that you feel off balance and need to hold something.

Safety Tip

Move slowly and with your breath in this sequence. Keep a microbend in the standing leg to protect your knee.

Ankle Sit/Toe Sit

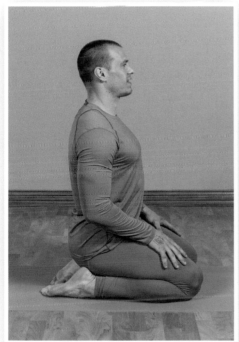

FIGURE 8.12a

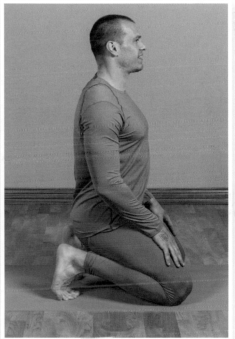

FIGURE 8.12b

Muscles

Abductor hallucis, extensor hallucis, extensor digitorum, Achilles tendon, adductor digiti minimi

1. Lower to your mat to hands and knees.

2. Uncurl your back toes, and sit back onto your heels, sitting up tall with your shoulders over your hips and your hands resting on your thighs (figure 8.12a).

3. After holding the ankle sit for 10 breaths, place your hands on the floor in front of your knees and lean forward to return to hands and knees.

(continued)

4. Curl your toes under, and sit back onto your heels (figure 8.12*b*). Sit up tall with your shoulders over your hips and your hands on your thighs.

5. Hold the position for 10 breaths. Repeat the sequence two more times.

Modification

Place a block standing tall in front of your knees, and place both hands on the block. This modification allows your shoulders and torso to be forward, taking some of the pressure off the feet.

Safety Tip

If your feet and ankles are very tight, do not hold this pose for the full 10 breaths; hold it for a breath or two, then switch. It's better to ease into this stretch and slowly build flexibility in your feet.

Eagle Pose

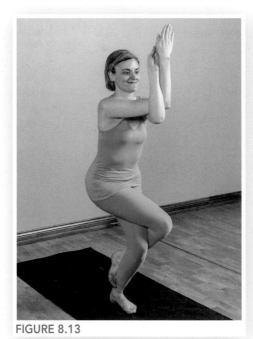

FIGURE 8.13

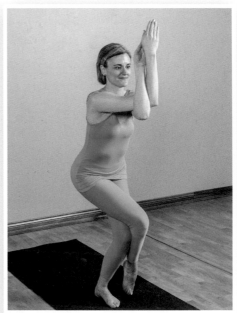

FIGURE 8.14 Eagle pose, modification.

Muscles

Flexor digitorum, soleus, gastrocnemius, Achilles tendon

1. Standing at the top of your mat, cross your right leg over your left thigh as you bend your left knee to a half chair pose.

2. Wrap your right foot behind your left ankle.

3. Reach your arms out to your sides, then bring your arms together and hook your left arm under your right elbow.

4. Bend both elbows, and wrap the palms together (figure 8.13).

5. Push your forearms forward, and lift your fingers to the ceiling.

6. Hold the pose for 5 to 10 breaths, and repeat it on the other side.

Modifications

If your foot does not wrap around your ankle, just rest the foot next to the ankle (figure 8.14). The same goes for the hands; if your palms don't meet, let the backs of your hands touch. If your balance is off today, use your right foot as a kickstand to help with your balance while in this pose.

Safety Tip

To help with balance, follow the modification of resting the foot next to the ankle as shown in figure 8.14.

Standing Big Toe Hold

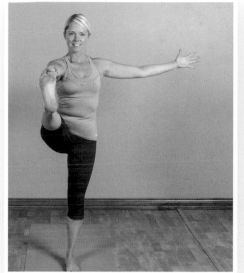

FIGURE 8.15a

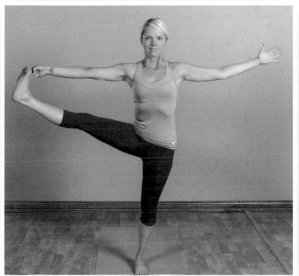

FIGURE 8.15b

Muscles

Gastrocnemius, soleus, peroneus longus and brevis, tibialis anterior, extensor hallucis, adductor hallucis, extensor digitorum, flexor digitorum, adductor digiti minimi, trochlea tali, flexor hallucis, tibialis posterior

1. Standing at the top of your mat, put your weight onto your left foot and pull your right knee to your chest.
2. Use the first two fingers of your right hand, and wrap them around your right big toe.
3. Stand tall as you straighten your right leg out in front of you, reaching your left arm out to your left side (figure 8.15a).
4. Slowly move your right leg to the right, keeping the leg long, and move your focal point to the left (figure 8.15b).
5. Slowly move your right leg back out in front of you.
6. Hold both positions for 5 breaths, then switch legs.

(continued)

Modifications

If your hamstrings are a bit tight, use a yoga strap so that you can stand tall and straighten your leg long (figure 8.16*a*). You can also stand next to a wall and place your left hand on the wall to help with your balance (figure 8.16*b*).

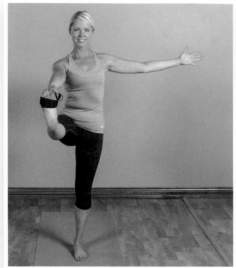

FIGURE 8.16*a* Standing big toe hold, modification with strap.

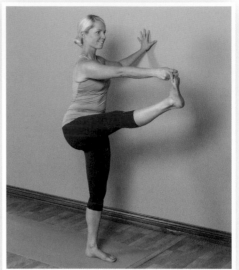

FIGURE 8.16*b* Standing big toe hold, modification next to wall.

Safety Tip

Follow the modification using the strap and the wall to help with both balance and tight hamstrings.

One-Legged Chair Pose

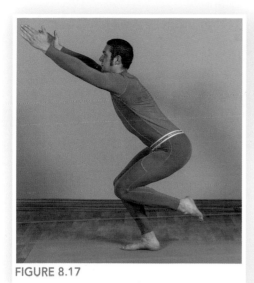

FIGURE 8.17

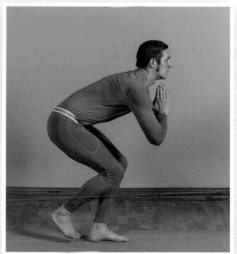

FIGURE 8.18 One-legged chair pose, modification.

Muscles

Flexor digitorum, soleus, gastrocnemius, Achilles tendon

1. Standing on your mat, bring your feet and knees together.
2. Bend both knees, and put your weight back onto your heels, squeezing your knees together as you sweep your arms up to the ceiling, tucking your tailbone under as you enter into chair pose.
3. Put your weight onto your right foot, and keep squeezing your knees together.
4. Deepen the bend in your left knee as you pull your left heel up to your left hip, keeping both knees squeezing together (figure 8.17).
5. Hold the pose for 10 to 15 breaths, then switch legs.

Modification

Bring your palms together in prayer in front of your chest. Instead of pulling your right heel up to your hip, just hover your foot a little off the floor (figure 8.18).

Safety Tip

Follow the modification to slowly ease into the balance.

Summary

The feet are the part of the human body used most every day. To keep them healthy, you have to take care of your feet and ankles. Keeping this part of the body strong, mobile, and loose will prevent sprains, ankle twists, and turf toe, and it will keep you strong and quick. Strength and flexibility go hand in hand for every athlete. Many sports require quick movements. Balance is a key quality for unexpected split-second body shifts.

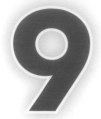

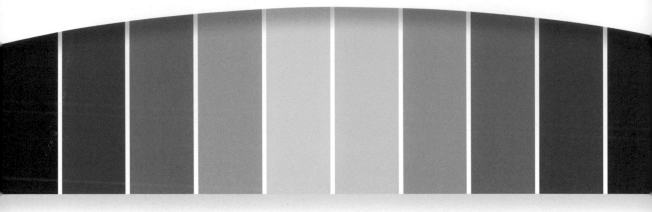

COOLING DOWN, MEDITATING, AND VISUALIZING: IN THE ZONE

This chapter focuses on the importance of the cool-down and a meditation practice for all athletes in all sports. Visualization is also a key component for focus and concentration on the field, court, or track. It is easy to get so caught up in the powerful aspects of athletics that you underestimate the physical importance of a cool-down and meditation practice for a sport or a yoga practice. After a rigorous workout or yoga practice the body needs a cool-down. This phase allows the body to slowly return to its natural resting state with ease. It is also why relaxation is so important at the end of any yoga practice. Meditation not only calms the nervous system but has many physical benefits as well. Staying calm and focused can help with performance on game day and even practices. This chapter begins with the cool-down from your yoga practice and eases into relaxation and meditation. Finally, it covers visualization for success.

Cool-Down

Just as in any workout, practice, or training session, a balanced yoga practice must always include a cool-down. A cool-down allows the body a smooth transition back to its resting state. It helps you to reduce your heart and breathing rates and gradually cool your body temperature, especially if you took your yoga practice to the next level and increased your heart rate.

Following are some simple stretches that are great for the end of your practice.

Cool-Down Stretches

1 Begin with cat/cow. Start on your hands and knees, aligning your hands under your shoulders and your knees under your hips. Inhale as you drop your belly and lift your chin and tailbone up toward the ceiling (figure 9.1a). Exhale as you tuck your chin to your chest, tuck your tailbone under, press into your palms to keep your arms straight, and arch your upper back toward the ceiling (figure 9.1b).

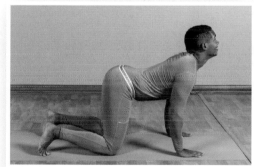
FIGURE 9.1a Cat/cow.

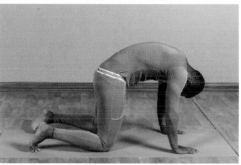
FIGURE 9.1b

2 After a few repetitions of cat/cow, moving with your breath, push back into child's pose. Bring your big toes together, and separate your knees. Move your hips back to your heels, relaxing your forehead to the floor. Walk your hands to the far right of your mat (figure 9.2a) and then to the far left of your mat (figure 9.2b).

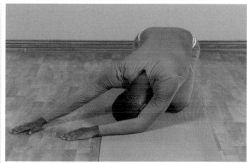
FIGURE 9.2a Child's pose.

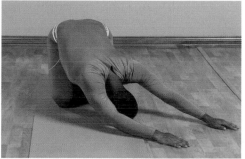
FIGURE 9.2b

3 Move into a seated spinal twist (figure 9.3). Sit on your mat, and straighten both legs in front of you. Bend your right knee into your chest, and plant your right foot on the mat. Plant your right hand on the mat behind your hips. Bend your left elbow, and cross your elbow to the outside of your right knee. Press your right palm firmly into the mat to lengthen your spine. Gently pull your left elbow into your right knee to twist. Keep the left leg long and your left foot flexed. Hold for 5 to 10 breaths. Switch sides.

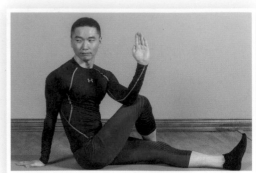

FIGURE 9.3 Seated spinal twist.

4 Move into a seated forward fold (figure 9.4). Straighten both legs in front of you. Rotate the legs in toward each other, and flex your feet so that your toes point toward the ceiling. Sit up tall, and reach both arms toward the ceiling. Hinging at your hips reach forward for your toes. Wrap your hands around your feet, and relax your head down to your shins.

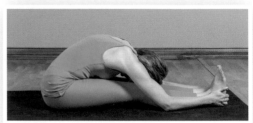

FIGURE 9.4 Seated forward fold.

5 Move into a head to knee pose (figure 9.5). Stretch both legs in front of you. Bring your left knee up to your chest and plant the left foot on the mat on the inside of your right thigh. Lower your left knee toward the ground. Sit tall, and reach both arms up to the ceiling. Fold forward, grabbing your right foot with both hands. Relax your head down to your right leg. Switch sides.

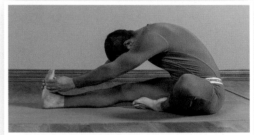

FIGURE 9.5 Head to knee pose.

6 Finish with a supine spinal twist with knees together (figure 9.6). Lie on your back, and pull both knees into your chest. Extend your arms out to your sides and down to the floor, palms down. Keep your knees and ankles together as you lower both legs to the right and look to the left. Switch to the other side.

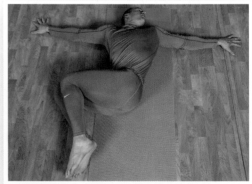

FIGURE 9.6 Supine spinal twist with knees together.

Relaxation Pose

At the end of every yoga practice, it is important to relax. Just as in a cool-down, relaxation helps to center your body while bringing it to its natural resting state. In Sanskrit, this pose is known as *savasana*, which literally means "corpse pose." In your yoga practice, you will find poses that you love and that feel great, but you may also find poses that are challenging and frustrating. In addition, sometimes in your practice your mind races, and you may feel heavy and not in the practice. People encounter these same types of challenges in fitness workouts, sport practices, and training sessions. A relaxation session allows your body and mind to stop at the end of your yoga practice, bringing stillness and calmness. In addition, it allows your heart rate to slow down and your breath to return to its natural flow and rhythm. You should stay in relaxation for as long as you can, but try to commit to 3 to 5 minutes or more.

To enter into relaxation, lie on your back, straighten your legs, and place your arms along your sides with your palms turned up. If you feel pain in your lower back with your legs straight, bend your knees with your feet on the mat or butterfly the knees apart. Close your eyes as you start to relax your whole body. To let go, start by relaxing your forehead. Soften your jaw as you relax your tongue down from the top of your mouth and separate your teeth. Relax your shoulders into the mat, allowing your arms to let go and roll open. Relax your back as you release any tension in your belly and chest. Feel your hips melt down into your mat as your legs and feet let go and roll apart. Quiet your mind of any thoughts or planning, and take this time to let go and enjoy, allowing yourself to drift into your relaxation.

Meditation

Meditation is spending time in quiet thought for spiritual or relaxation purposes. Meditation has many benefits that help the physical body and the mental body (the mind). In today's society, one of the most common issues affecting people is stress. Stress can harm the physical body and the mind. While in meditation, you often focus on your breathing. Taking just three deep breaths can help calm the nervous system and relax the mind as it brings fresh oxygen into the body's systems and your cells. Taking even a minute to relax your mind on one simple thought or sound helps to calm the mind.

High stress can cause high blood pressure. When people are stressed, they tend to neglect their bodies and fall into unhealthy habits. Stress is exhausting and can wear heavy on the mind. If you don't let go of your day at bedtime, it can lead to poor sleeping patterns. Poor sleep can lead

KEIFER SYKES

University of Wisconsin—Green Bay, Austin Spurs, Guard

Yoga has helped me benefit in a number of ways in basketball. Yoga more than anything has helped me increase my consciousness of focus, which helps me stay connected with my mind throughout the duration of an emotional game. I love the meditation and relaxation aspects of yoga, so before the games I like to meditate on the task that I have to complete during the games. Oftentimes I'm able to visualize an effective performance of the game, which helps me get relaxed, more controlled, and prepared to compete.

to feeling tired or sluggish the following day, which can then make it very easy to reach for high-sugar foods and drinks for a short-term energy rush. In turn, when the sugars have metabolized, you encounter the sugar crash that makes you even more sluggish and tired. At this point, any motivation to exercise is gone, causing a downward spiral of events that in time leads to high blood pressure. Meditation is a great start to help relax your mind and find calm in your life, which can help prevent the stress spiral. Lastly, it is important to take some time for yourself each day; more specifically, take some time to stop and let go of thoughts or planning, and focus on one thing. With time and practice, this calm focus can help to reduce blood pressure.

Anxiety is common in today's fast-paced society. Life places many demands on people, and too often they allow themselves to take on too much. When symptoms of anxiety arise, such as shortness of breath and tightening in the chest, you can feel vulnerable and withdrawn. With time and practice sitting in meditation, you will build the awareness of how to handle your anxiety when the moment arises. Similar to when beginning meditation, close your eyes, bringing your awareness to your breath. Focus on deep, long, and slow inhalations and exhalations for as many rounds as you need to help you relax. Meditation is a great tool to help calm yourself during unexpected and unwanted moments of anxiety.

Here is a simple meditation exercise to help you get started:

- Sit or lie down somewhere comfortable for you, such as a chair, couch, yoga mat, or meditation bolster.
- Close your eyes.
- Relax your whole body.
- Quiet your mind for a moment, and breathe naturally.
- Focus on your body while you breathe. Keeping your awareness on your body, begin to relax more as you let thoughts pass by. If your mind begins to wander, refocus on your body and your natural breathing.
- Practice this technique for 1 minute at a time, and try to add another minute each time you practice.

When you are ready to explore meditation a bit further, try the following techniques. See what works best for you.

GUIDED MEDITATION

This type of meditation guides you with audio from your phone, television, or computer, and it can be one of the easiest ways to meditate. This technique guides you into a state of deep relaxation by a prerecorded voice that walks you step by step through your daily meditation practice. As the speaker guides you into your meditation, he or she uses visualization and imaging techniques to suggest positive personal changes to your daily life. During this meditation, you are led into a deep state of relaxation while listening to positive affirmations or suggestions. Guided meditation allows you to clear your mind of clutter and unwanted thoughts. It adds positive, inspiring thoughts for great personal changes, which can lead to deep inner peace and stillness.

CONCENTRATION MEDITATION

This technique allows you to focus on only one thing. This one thing can be anything from focusing on your breathing, staring at a candle, or repeating one word over and over in your head. If your mind drifts away, bring your attention back to your object or phrase where you left it. While focusing on your breathing, notice the length in each breath you take. Try counting the length of time it takes you to take in a smooth, slow, long inhalation, then count the length of time on your exhalation. In time and with practice, you will notice that your count will be longer for each inhalation and each exhalation.

Lighting a candle and placing it on a nearby table or the floor can also aid you with your concentration meditation. Sit comfortably, and relax your whole body. Take your gaze to the candle and just stare at the candle, letting all thoughts pass by. Focus on the flame changing shape and height.

The last option for concentration meditation is repeating one word or a sentence over and over in your head. Be comfortable in your space, and close your eyes. Choose a word or sentence that is positive and inspiring to you. Take a few breaths, and start to repeat that word or sentence in your head calmly and slowly. As you repeat it in your head, thoughts or planning will trickle in, but let them go immediately and return to your word or sentence. As you practice more often, try to sit longer each time. With practice you will find calm and ease, and you will add enhanced focus to your concentration, allowing you to let go of random thoughts more easily.

WALKING MEDITATION

Walking meditation can be great for people who have high-stress jobs. Choose a path or trail that is quiet and relaxing to you. Find a comfortable, moderate walking pace that is not strenuous. Start to focus on your feet and each step you take. Notice when each heel touches the ground and the roll of the foot as you take each stride forward. Take note of the back foot as the heel lifts and the roll of the foot forward. As you take each step, feel the motion of your feet and the movement each foot takes. Be aware of details such as the rubbing of your socks on your skin, the tightness in your ankles, or the calmness of your movement. Take in the sounds that surround you on this walk, such as the leaves in the wind, birds chirping, or the sounds your feet make on each step. Be aware of your surroundings by noticing the vibrant colors of the trees, grasses, or sky, and take it all in at that moment. Take in deep breaths as your body continues to move. This simple technique allows your body to be moving and is considered a mild form of exercise. Walking meditation gets your blood flowing through your body while at the same time relaxing your mind and body.

Many other meditation techniques can be incorporated into your practice. There is no right or wrong way to meditate; it's all about relaxing the mind and taking time for you to relax and rejuvenate, resulting in a calm, centered lifestyle.

Visualization

Athletes' bodies are trained for their positions, but they also need to apply their minds to their positions and to game day. They must prepare their minds as well as their bodies. Therefore, the sequence for guided visualization in this book is set for athletes' minds to succeed. For example, a football player may picture game day like this: putting on his uniform, walking through the tunnel onto the field, and seeing himself make the game-winning play. This application of yoga techniques to the specific needs of athletes is what makes the practice presented in this book different, effective, and worth trying.

Athletes train their bodies hard and push their bodies beyond the limit, but what about their minds? You should ask yourself this question when training for an event or sport. The mind is a powerful tool. You may not expect it, but the mind is just as strong, if not stronger, than your physical body. Learning to train your mind is just as important as training your physical body. Visualization is a great tool to train your mind for your sport. As the saying goes, what you put your mind to, you will achieve.

Visualization is a natural process of harnessing the power of your mind and the power of thoughts. This mental technique uses deep thought and imagination to make dreams and goals come true. One way to use visualization using this kind of deep thought can be similar to daydreaming. Daydreaming is allowing yourself to drift away in your vision of yourself in a dream or goal that you want to achieve. You are mentally putting yourself in the moment you are wishing for. Daydreaming can happen while on the computer, while watching TV, or while standing around to check out at a store. Other ways to visualize can be similar to meditation, such as sitting or lying comfortably and focusing only on your vision and the sequence in which you want to see things happen, and repeating this vision over and over. Either of these options is the start to your visualization.

Everyone should use visualization in daily life. You may be looking to have success in your career, make more money, improve your life, find love, or for certain events to happen. Visualization applies to everyone who has goals and wishes. You have to put your mind to your wish or goal and allow the natural mental laws to do their job.

To make visualization work, give yourself some time alone anywhere that is comfortable and relaxing to you. Either close your eyes or stare off at a distance, and decide what your vision will be. See yourself in this vison going through each step or task needed to achieve the end result. Your vision may have you making the winning shot, kick, tackle, or throw, achieving a running pace, and so on. Keep repeating this image or task in your head, and feel the feelings and emotions of the success from your vision in your heart. Through time and by repeating this image, you are conditioning yourself to follow through with this task. When this vision comes true it will feel familiar, reducing your nerves in that moment, making you more likely to succeed.

When applying these mental thoughts and feelings to your visualizations, you are creating a mental workout. You start to feel your heart race and the increased rhythm in your breathing. Your blood races through your veins as it would while playing the sport. A jolt of tingling zips through your body from the excitement of a good play or a win. Having these physical feelings while you are focusing on your visualization stimulates your sympathetic nervous system, creating a fight-or-flight response. These feelings, emotions, and physical reactions are the same ones you will have when you live out your vision.

Linking your mind with your emotions is your mental workout, which then enhances your vision, allowing it to come true. Using your visions to create success can enhance your motivation to practice harder and not give up. In addition, your visions will give you the confidence to perform in the critical moments of your sport. Just as in the physical part of a sport, things don't always work out. The same thing can happen with visualizations. You may mentally prep for your plays; however, they may not come to fruition. Don't give up! Keep working on your visions, have patience and faith, and know that results will start to happen when they are supposed to happen for you.

Following is one of the visualizations that I have used when working with professional athletes. It is basic, but simple enough to understand and build on for each athlete. This simple technique guided players to come up with their own visualization to help them work and play harder on the field:

Just off preseason I started to push the mental aspect of the game on the players, giving simple examples to guide them to the direction of visualization. At the end of class I would have them lie down comfortably on their backs, close their eyes, and follow my instructions visually in their heads. We would start with our walkthrough of gearing up on game day. Next I would have them see themselves walking through the tunnel and onto the field, hearing the whole stadium erupting with loud cheers and exciting yelling. We would follow our vision walking onto the field and getting into their positon getting ready for a play. Next I would lead them to their actual play on the field and the feelings they had while envisioning being on the field. From here, I wanted each athlete to find the exact play, moment, or action he felt would be his winning visualization. Once each player found the play he wanted, one that was right for him, I told him to replay that moment over and over in his head, to see himself making the play and hearing the sounds, to experience the feelings and emotions radiating in his chest and gut, to keep repeating all of this as often as possible.

Daydream or visualize this vision while driving to work, sitting at home in silence, or at lunch.

TRAMON WILLIAMS
NFL Cornerback

I was introduced to visualization by Ryanne in our yoga sessions. We would typically start off the class with an intense session of yoga, and toward the end of the session she would give us a couple of different options of relaxation; visualization was one of the options. I found visualization relaxing, taking me to a place of peace, knowledge, and even a place of preparation. As I got more experienced with visualizing through working with Ryanne, it began to naturally happen. As I would lie down in bed and prepare for sleep, I would naturally visualize something that was on my mind. Even when I was well awake, I still had the capabilities to visualize what I needed at the time. (Some may say this is daydreaming. I feel that when you are daydreaming you are having a random dream, but I seemed to go where I wanted to go with these visions.) It began to help me on the football field, and it even helped with everyday life. As I would begin preparing for my opponents I naturally found myself visualizing about certain plays, situations, certain moments in the game that I was prepping for physically, but I was now doing the same thing from a mental standpoint. It was like I would bring that moment alive before I would ever truly live out that moment. I could see myself making those plays that I've studied on film and even prepared for all week at practice. Let me be the first to say that during the week of practice I may get beat on some of those same plays, situations, and moments that I see visually. Visualization took me to a place on the field where no moment was too big for me. I am totally focused and prepared. I am never underprepared mentally, because my mind is always working, even when I am relaxing. That's a powerful skill to have if you learn how to use it.

Summary

This chapter has highlighted all of the benefits of a cool-down, relaxation and meditation practice, and visualization. The chapter provided some examples from which you can choose to work best for you and your training. Staying calm and in the moment adds to sport performance and overall well-being.

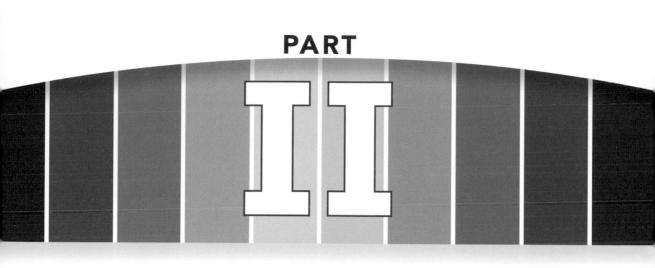

PART

II

Poses
for Sport-Specific
Performance

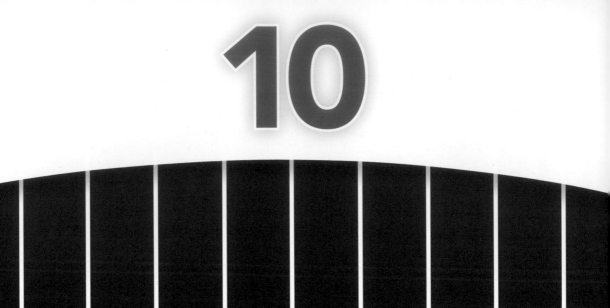

FOOTBALL: STRETCHES FOR EVERY POSITION

American football includes many positions, and each requires different stretches to maximize performance. This chapter outlines the poses that all football players need to help prevent injuries and enhance their performance on the field. Football injuries range from legs and ankles up through shoulders and arms. Focusing on these specific areas will decrease the chances of injury, as well as increase speed and flexibility, both of which will help when blocking, tackling, or extending for the ball. In addition to these specific areas, football players should take the time to stretch the whole body instead of just one part of the body to help in other motions used on the field. Each play is different and requires split-second movements that may require subtle areas of the body usually not associated with playing football. An example of such an area is the ankles. Most players focus most stretching on the large muscles. Ankle sit/toe sit has a great benefit to preventing ankle rolling, sprains, and even turf toe. Yoga can help keep these areas become flexible and adaptable.

The poses presented for this sport are for every position and for the whole body. Each pose was chosen to target areas football players generally have tightness in or areas that are injury prone. Take the time to hold each pose for 10 to 20 breaths or longer. Try to relax while holding the pose instead of fighting the stretch. Repeat a side that seems tighter, and hold it longer. Following these guidelines will help you stay loose, mobile, and ready for your next game.

Ankle Sit/Toe Sit

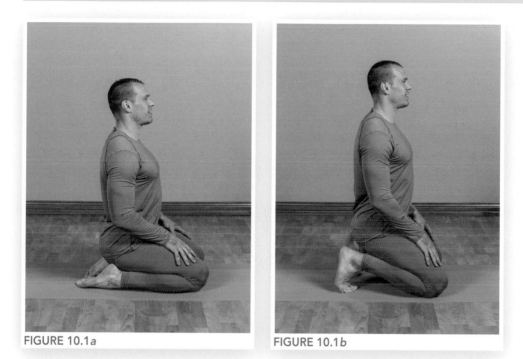

FIGURE 10.1a

FIGURE 10.1b

Whether you play on natural or artificial turf, the feet take a pounding during football games or practice. The ankle sit/toe sit sequence stretches the small muscles of the feet to provide relief and increase flexibility of the ankles. From downward-facing dog pose, bend both knees and lower to your hands and knees. Keep your toes curled under, and walk your hands back to your knees as you slowly take your hips to your heels. Lift your chest, aligning your shoulders over your hips. Sit tall; you have moved into toe sit (figure 10.1a). Next, walk your hands forward to return to your hands and knees. Uncurl your toes, and again walk your hands back to your knees. Sit on your heels; you have moved into ankle sit (figure 10.1b). Hold each pose for 10 to 20 breaths.

Pyramid Pose With Block

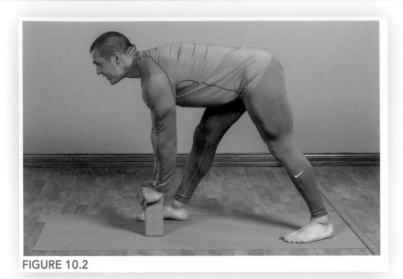

FIGURE 10.2

The explosive movements and speed required on the football field cause tight hamstrings in football players, and consequently hamstring pulls and strains are common in these athletes. Holding pyramid pose is key for flexibility in the hamstrings, which helps prevent injury. From downward-facing dog pose, step your right foot behind your right wrist. Hop your left foot a step forward and a step to the left, placing both feet flat on the mat and hip-width apart. Place a yoga block standing tall on the inside of your right foot. Place both hands on the block, keeping your arms straight, shoulders relaxed away from your ears, and spine long. Press into your right foot to straighten your right leg and to square your hips to the top of your mat (figure 10.2). You have moved into pyramid pose with a block.

Bow Pose

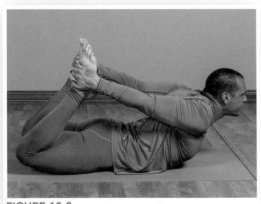

FIGURE 10.3

Football players tend to hunch forward in blocking or running for faster speed on the field. Bow pose not only counters that hunching by stretching and opening up the chest and shoulders, but it's also a great stretch for the low back and the front of the body, such as hip flexors and quadriceps. Lie on your belly. Lengthen both arms down along your sides. Bend both knees, and reach back for your ankles. Press your feet back into your hands, lifting your feet (figure 10.3). At the same time, pull your chest forward, maintaining a long spine and not sinking into your low back. Keep your gaze forward as you move into bow pose. A modification to this pose would be to take upward facing dog.

Warrior III Pose With Leg Movement

Balance is key in football. Players play on uneven ground and make split-second moves that sometimes require them to balance in interesting ways at a moment's notice. Warrior III pose with leg movement practices balance at all angles to prepare a player for such moves. From downward-facing dog pose, step your right foot forward between your hands and come to balance on your right leg; your torso and left leg are parallel to the floor. Reach your arms out to help with balance (figure 10.4a). Bend your left leg to your chest and come up to standing, balancing on your right leg (figure 10.4b). Straighten your left leg in front of you (figure 10.4c). Keeping your left leg high, slowly circle your left leg out to the left and back behind you, bringing you into warrior III. Slowly repeat this motion 3 to 5 times, then switch sides. A modification to this pose will be to hold warrior III pose instead of adding the movement. Use a block for the hands to help if your balance is off.

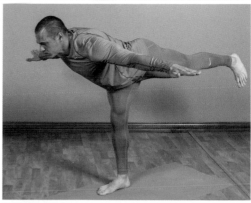

FIGURE 10.4a

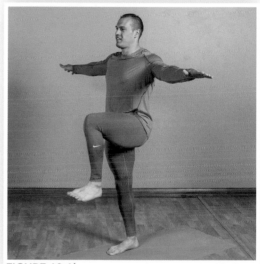

FIGURE 10.4b

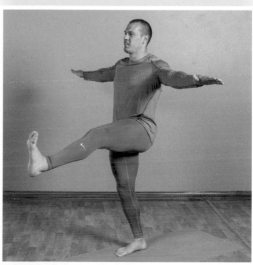

FIGURE 10.4c

185

High Lunge Pose With Hands on Floor

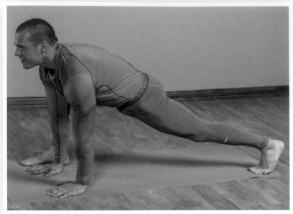

FIGURE 10.5

The quadriceps are big muscles that are important for running, jumping, and squatting, motions largely used in every position in football. High lunge pose with hands on floor will help lengthen the quadriceps and hip flexors. From downward-facing dog pose, step your right foot forward between your hands, keeping your left knee off the mat. Place both hands on the mat on the inside of your right foot, and walk your right foot to the right edge of your mat. Press both hands down into the mat, keeping your arms straight and your shoulders relaxed away from your shoulders. Bend your right knee forward as you push your left heel back, allowing your hips to sink toward the mat (figure 10.5). Keep lifting your chest.

Pigeon Pose to T.W. Side Pigeon Pose

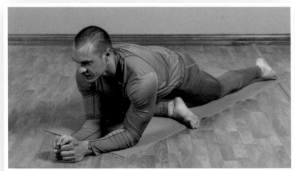

FIGURE 10.6a

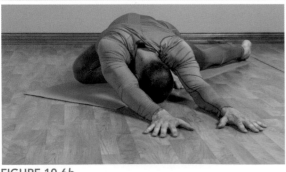

FIGURE 10.6b

Football players need to quickly perform lateral movements on the field. Pigeon pose to T.W. side pigeon pose targets the muscles needed for quick lateral movements on the field. From downward-facing dog pose, bend your right knee to your chest and place your right knee on the mat behind your right hand. Relax your left knee to the mat, and walk your left leg back as you shift your hips back. Square your hips to the mat, and walk down to your forearms. Separate your elbows, and lower to the floor (figure 10.6a). Hold the pose for 5 breaths. Walk your forearms to the left side of your mat as you push your right hip back. Reach your right arm out to the left side of the room, and relax your head, bowing down (figure 10.6b).

Shoulder Rotation With Strap

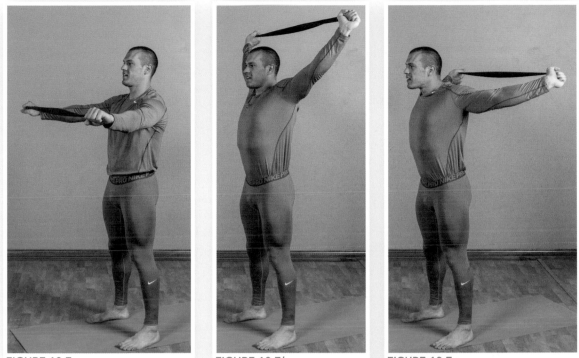

FIGURE 10.7*a*

FIGURE 10.7*b*

FIGURE 10.7*c*

Players in all positions greatly benefit from the shoulder rotation with strap. This exercise helps stretch the muscles used when reaching for a block or to catch a pass at any angle of the arm rotation or when throwing the football at high speed or height down the field. Stand and hold a strap in both hands; hands are more than shoulder-width apart and arms are straightened in front of you (figure 10.7*a*). Lift your arms up over your head (figure 10.7*b*), and allow your arms to fall behind you (figure 10.7*c*). Separate your hands along the strap enough to allow your arms to fall behind you. Slowly lift the arms back up and in front of you. Follow this motion, walking the hands in closer together once the shoulders loosen up.

Knee to Elbow

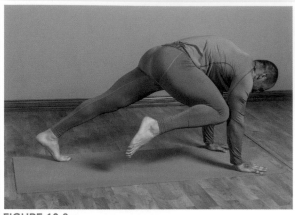

FIGURE 10.8*a*

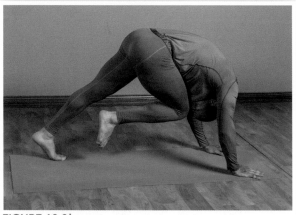

FIGURE 10.8*b*

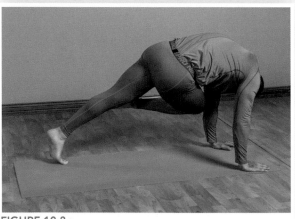

FIGURE 10.8*c*

A strong core powers all movements on the field for speed, agility, and strength. This variation of plank pose works the core. Starting from downward-facing dog pose, lift your right leg to the ceiling to three-legged downward-facing dog pose. Bend your right knee, and shift forward to plank pose, aligning your shoulders over your wrists and taking your right knee to your right elbow (figure 10.8*a*) and squeezing your core. Move back to three-legged downward-facing dog pose. Bend your right knee and shift forward to plank pose, bringing your right knee to your nose (figure 10.8*b*). Go back to three-legged downward-facing dog pose. Bend your right knee and shift forward to plank pose, bringing your right knee to your left elbow (figure 10.8*c*). Finish in downward-facing dog pose. Repeat the sequence using the left leg.

Half Crisscross Pose

An open and mobile shoulder can prevent shoulder injury and even protect the biceps and triceps, preventing any muscle tears or pulling. Lie on your abdomen, and come up to your forearms, aligning your elbows under your shoulders. Turning your right palm faceup, slide your right arm behind your left elbow, reaching out to your left. Extend your left arm forward as you lower your chest to the floor (figure 10.9). Lower your left armpit toward the floor. Come back to your starting position, then repeat the pose on the left side.

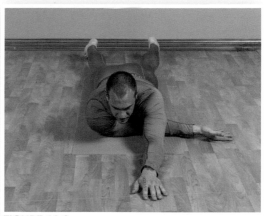

FIGURE 10.9

Supine Revolving Big Toe Hold With Strap

In football, running and other quick, multidirectional movements on uneven ground provoke tightness in the hips. Supine revolved big toe hold gives a player the mobility and flexibility needed to stay quick on the field. Lie supine (on your back). Grab a yoga strap. Place the strap around the ball of your right foot, and straighten your right leg up to the ceiling. Take both ends of the strap in your right hand, and lower your right leg to the right as you look to your left (figure 10.10a). Slowly take the right leg back up. Take both ends of the strap in your left hand, and lower your right leg to your left (figure 10.10b) as close to the floor as you like. Look to your right. Roll your right hip forward, and keep pushing through your right heel to keep your leg long. Switch legs.

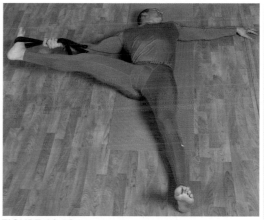

FIGURE 10.10a

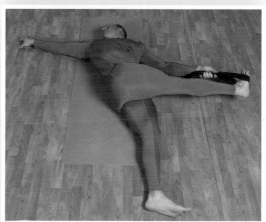

FIGURE 10.10b

Seated Half Neck Roll

Football helmets are lighter than they use to be, but anytime you start a new season, the helmets create tightness and stiffness in the neck. Seated neck roll is an easy yet efficient way to keep the neck loose and mobile. Sit up tall with your shoulders relaxed away from your ears. Take your chin to your chest, and slowly roll your right ear to your right shoulder (figure 10.11a). Continue to roll your head forward to your chest and then over to your left shoulder (figure 10.11b). Move slowly from one shoulder to the other. Gently move your head to center, and lift it. Relax your head back, lifting your chin up (figure 10.11c). Continue rolling the head from right shoulder to left shoulder.

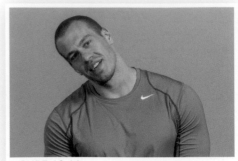

FIGURE 10.11a

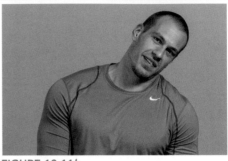

FIGURE 10.11b

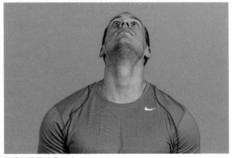

FIGURE 10.11c

Summary

All the poses in this chapter have been used on professional football players, and each player has greatly benefitted from them. No player wants to miss a game because of an injury, so taking the time to use each pose as part of your stretch routine will help your body stay loose, mobile and ready for game day.

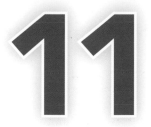

11

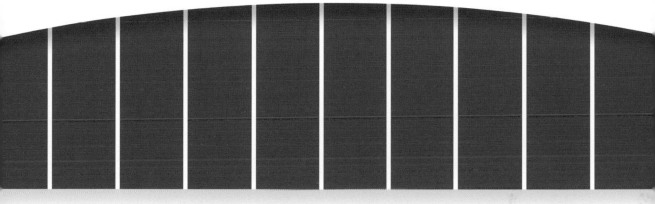

RUNNING: MORE THAN LEGS

Runners often think that to be top performers, they need to focus only on their legs. However, runners also need to increase shoulder mobility, core strength, and flexibility in the spine, hips, and related connective tissues. The arms provide momentum as they swing forward and back. This repetitive motion can create tightness in the shoulders. The hamstrings and quadriceps are a runner's constant power force in short and long runs. The repetitive motion and forward-leaning posture in running make it a physically demanding sport, so runners must take good care of their bodies. To prevent injury from tight muscles, runners need a stretching routine. The poses in this chapter address all the needs of runners. They also decrease muscle recovery time, allowing runners to continue their training more easily. During each stretch, try to hold each pose for 5 to 10 breaths and switch sides.

Plank Pose With IT Band Stretch

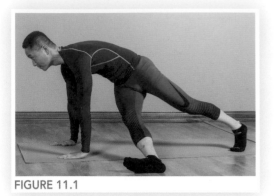

FIGURE 11.1

One of the most common sites of tightness or injury from the constant pounding on cement is the IT band. A simple stretch such as plank pose with IT band stretch will decrease that irritating achiness in the IT band and keep you away from IT band injury. From plank pose, bend your right knee to your chest. Flexing your right foot, straighten your right leg to the left, lowering your foot to the floor. Eventually work toward getting your toes to line up with your fingers (figure 11.1). Hook your right hip under as you lengthen forward through your collarbones.

Seated Forward Fold

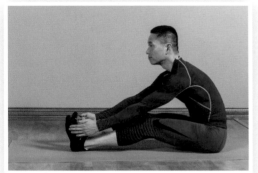

FIGURE 11.2

Runners' hamstrings are quick to tighten up, and tight hamstrings can lead to low-back pain. Seated forward fold will keep your hamstrings loose and flexible. Sit on your mat, and straighten both legs out in front of you. Bring them together, keeping your feet flexed. Walk your hands down your legs, reaching for your feet, and wrap your hands around your feet. Bend your elbows out to the sides to lengthen your spine forward (figure 11.2). Use a yoga strap around your feet and bend at your knees slightly for a hamstring stretch if you cannot touch your feet.

Low Lunge Pose

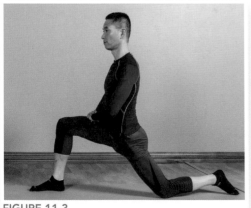

FIGURE 11.3

Staying balanced is key for runners to keep an even pace when training. The quadriceps is an important muscle group needed for running, and low lunge quadriceps variation will stretch the quadriceps to keep the legs balanced. Start in downward-facing dog pose. Step your right foot forward between your hands, and lower your left knee to the mat. Place both hands on your right thigh to lift your torso as you lunge forward (figure 11.3). Next, shift your hips back slightly as you bend your left knee. Lunge forward again. Switch legs.

Boat Pose to Half Boat Pose

A strong core not only protects the back but also helps with posture, which then gives a runner a better pace and time. Sit on your mat with both knees bent and feet planted on the mat, parallel to each other. Wrap your hands around your hamstrings, and sit tall. Lean your torso back and lift your feet off the mat, balancing on your sitting bones. Release your hands, turning your palms faceup (figure 11.4a). Straighten your legs so that you are in a V-shaped position; this is boat pose. Slowly lower your torso and legs to hover above the ground in half boat pose on your exhale (figure 11.4b), and lift back up to boat pose as you inhale. Perform 5 to 10 repetitions for two sets.

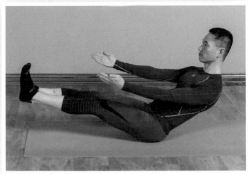

FIGURE 11.4a

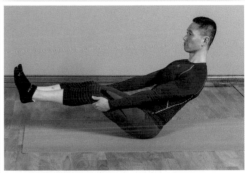

FIGURE 11.4b

Seated Spinal Twist

When running, the body's focus is forward and little lateral movement or torso turning occur. Seated spinal twist helps to ease the side-body and mid-back stiffness. Sit and extend both legs out in front of you. Bend your right knee to your chest, and plant your right foot on the mat on the outside of your left thigh. Plant your right hand on the floor behind your hips. Wrap your left arm around your right knee. Press into your right palm to lengthen your spine up, and twist your torso to your right (figure 11.5). Switch sides.

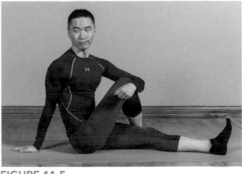

FIGURE 11.5

Runner's Back Lunge Pose

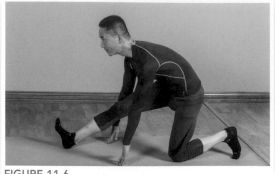

FIGURE 11.6

Keeping the hamstrings loose and flexible with runner's back lunge helps to keep runners free of pain and injury. Start in a low lunge pose with your right foot forward. Place both hands on the mat on each side of your right foot. Curl your left toes under, and shift your hips back toward your left foot. Go back only until your right leg straightens. Flex your right foot, and walk both hands forward (figure 11.6). Look forward to lengthen your spine, and hook your right hip under. Switch sides.

Bridge Pose

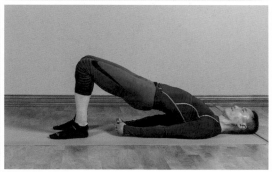

FIGURE 11.7

Repetitive pounding on cement while running can create tension in the back. Being in a backbend such as bridge pose can ease tense muscles. Lie on your back. Bend both knees, and plant your feet on the mat hip-width apart. Extend both arms down along your sides, and walk your heels to your fingertips. Pressing your feet down into your mat, lift your hips. Push your knees forward, lifting your chest up to your chin to lengthen your spine. Walk your shoulders under you and interlace your fingers, lowering your forearms to the mat (figure 11.7).

Open Chest Pose

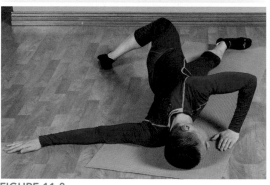

FIGURE 11.8

Runners tend to lean the torso forward while running. This forward-leaning posture allows the shoulders to gradually drop forward, causing tightness in the chest and shoulders. Open chest pose helps to broaden the space in the chest and the front of the shoulders, thus creating a feeling of openness. Lie on your belly. Turn your head to look to your right, and reach your right arm directly out of your right shoulder with your palm facing down. Then look to your left, relaxing your head on your mat as you place your left palm under your left shoulder. Bend your left knee, then lift your left thigh off the mat as you flip your left leg behind your right leg, planting your left foot on the mat (figure 11.8). Press your left palm into your mat to turn your left shoulder back and deepen the stretch. Switch sides.

Standing Big Toe Hold

Runners are faced with uneven ground and elements of weather that will challenge their balance. Standing big toe hold trains the control a runner needs for these elements of nature. Stand at the top of your mat. Lean your weight onto your left foot. Bend your right knee, and bring it up to your chest. Hook your right index finger and middle finger around the big toe of your right foot; the fingers are between the big toe and second toe and gripping so that you can externally rotate the right shoulder. Extend your right foot forward in front of you, straightening your right leg; your left arm is reaching out to the left shoulder height, or your left hand is resting on a wall for support (figure 11.9). Stand tall, and slowly move your right leg to your right side as you open the left arm out to the left with the hand at shoulder height. Look to your left. Switch legs.

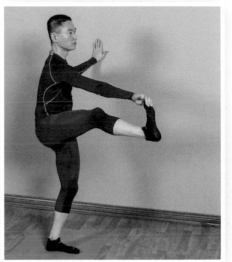

FIGURE 11.9

Seated Cow Face Pose

Running creates repetitive motion in the hips. Seated cow face pose eases the tightness in the outer hips that is associated with running. Sit on your mat with both legs lengthened in front of you. Bend your right knee to your chest, and cross your right leg over your left leg, stacking your knees. Bend your bottom leg, and slide your left foot next to your right hip. Walk your hands forward as you rest your chest on your right inner thigh and place your chin to your right knee (figure 11.10). Switch legs.

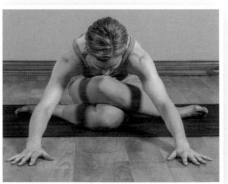

FIGURE 11.10

Side-Bending Low Lunge Pose

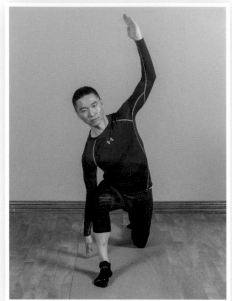

FIGURE 11.11

The quadriceps is one of the most used muscle groups in running, so keeping the quadriceps loose is key for performance and injury prevention. Side-bending lunge pose stretches the quadriceps. From downward-facing dog pose, step your right foot forward between your hands and lower your left knee to the floor in a low lunge. Place both hands on your right thigh, and lunge your hips forward. Relax your right arm down along your side, and reach your left arm to the ceiling. Start to lean your torso to your right, reaching your right arm down toward or onto the floor. Reach your left arm up and slightly back to open your chest, keeping your hips in a low lunge position (figure 11.11). Switch sides.

Summary

To have a quality run, you need your whole body to function well. The legs drive you forward, but the upper body aids in momentum and speed. This chapter has targeted all aspects a runner needs to stay loose, maintain a strong core, and therefore aid in a faster, less injury-prone run.

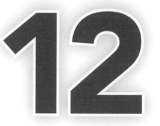

12

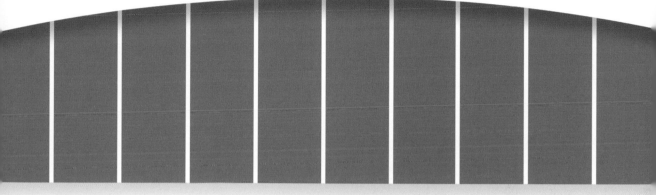

SOCCER: BRING BALANCE TO THE WORKOUT

The most common injuries that soccer players experience occur in the knees and ankles. Sprains and strains of the lower extremities are common in soccer and range in severity. Other common injuries that are less severe include groin pulls, thigh and calf strains, shin splints, Achilles tendinitis, and patellar tendinitis. Such injuries can be reduced by simply stretching the hamstrings, quadriceps, inner thighs, and calves. In addition, soccer players need balance work to make sure their ankles are strong and to improve split-second decisions and movements on the field. Soccer players also get tight in the upper torso from using their arms to build momentum while running and jumping quickly. Yoga bolsters endurance and improves joint strength through a low-impact routine. The poses in this chapter address all of these issues. Hold each pose for 5 to 10 breaths and switch sides.

Half Squat Pose

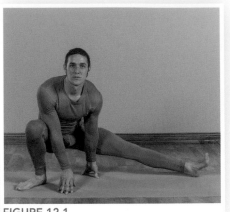

FIGURE 12.1

Soccer players need to be fast and make split-second movements on the field. Half squat pose keeps players loose in the inner thighs for speed and quick, explosive movements needed on the field. Stand at the top of your mat. Step your left foot back, and turn your right foot to the left so that you are standing with your legs wide. Turn your toes out slightly so that your feet are not parallel to each other. Fold forward, and place your hands on the mat. Bend your right knee, then walk your hands to your right foot as your left leg straightens and your left toes point up to the ceiling (figure 12.1). Keeping your right heel on the mat, sink your hips and lift your chest. Switch legs.

King Pigeon Pose

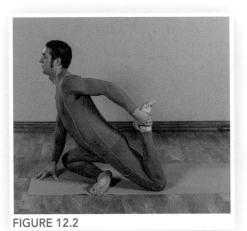

FIGURE 12.2

Soccer involves a lot of quick bursts; lateral, backward, and forward running; and fast, quick stops. All these moves require strong quadriceps muscles to keep movement fluid and fast. From downward-facing dog pose, bend your right knee to your chest, then place your right knee behind your right wrist. Lower your left knee to the floor. Walk your right foot up toward your left hand and lengthen your left leg back, shifting your hips back and down toward the mat. Bend your left knee, and reach back with your left hand for your left foot. Square your hips and shoulders with the front of your mat as you gently pull your left foot toward your left hip (figure 12.2). Switch legs.

Sugar Cane Pose

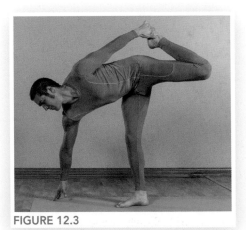

FIGURE 12.3

Outdoor soccer fields can feature uneven ground. During this fast sport, a player needs to be ready for any move on the field. Sugar cane pose trains the skill of balance, which can enhance strength in the ankles and feet. Starting from downward-facing dog pose, step your right foot forward between your hands and reach your right arm forward and slightly to the right. Lift up to balance on your right foot, keeping your right fingertips on the floor under your right shoulder. Reach your left arm up to the ceiling, and lengthen your left leg back to hip height. Bend your left leg, and wrap your left hand around your left foot (figure 12.3). Press your left foot into your left hand, opening your chest and shoulders as you maintain balance. Switch sides.

Puppy Pose Variation

While a soccer player's greatest assets are her legs, mobility of the upper body can help increase speed and jumping height. This puppy pose variation using two blocks loosens the shoulders and improves mobility for adding speed and height. Come to your hands and knees. Place two blocks at the top of your mat, side by side with an inch (about 2.5 cm) between the blocks. Place your right elbow on top of the block on your right and the same with your left elbow on the block to your left. Bring your palms together, and walk your knees back to lower your triceps to the blocks. Relax your head and chest toward the floor between your upper arms. Bend your elbows, and place your thumbs to your upper back (figure 12.4).

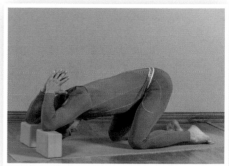

FIGURE 12.4

Windshield Wipers

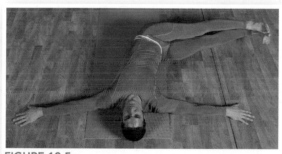

FIGURE 12.5*a*

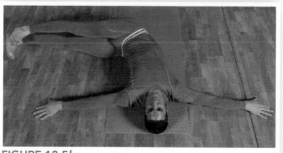

FIGURE 12.5*b*

The twists and turns in soccer require a strong core. Windshield wiper movements strengthen the core as the legs move side to side. Lie on your back. Reach both arms out and away from the shoulders, placing your palms facedown. Bend both knees up to your chest, and straighten your legs to the ceiling. Press your low back into the mat, and squeeze your core as you lower both legs to the right to hover over the ground (figure 12.5*a*). Slowly bring both legs back up to center, and continue to take the legs to the left to hover over the ground (figure 12.5*b*). Slowly move your legs side to side.

Triangle Pose

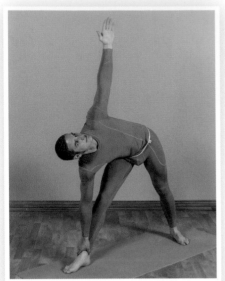

FIGURE 12.6

A player's body must be balanced to stay injury free. Given that the legs are the biggest asset to a soccer player, keeping the hamstrings loose and injury free is important. Triangle pose provides the best hamstring stretch for soccer players. Starting in downward-facing dog pose, step your right foot forward between your hands and lift your torso to standing. Align your right heel with your back foot arch. Angle your back heel back slightly. Turning your left hip forward a little, reach your right arm forward to the front of the room. Lean your torso forward as you reach for the front of the room and push your right hip back. Reach until you feel a stretch in your right hamstrings. Then relax your right arm down to your right shin or ankle. Reach your left arm up to the ceiling, stacking your shoulders (figure 12.6). Switch sides.

Prone Spinal Twist

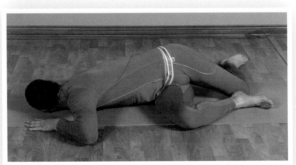

FIGURE 12.7

The legs do most of the work in soccer, but the upper body contributes, too. Full prone spinal twist gives the upper body a great stretch to ease up any tense and tight muscles. Sit on your mat and bend your knees, planting your feet mat-width apart. Place both hands on the ground behind you. Lower both legs to the ground on your right. Place your left hand next to your right hand to shift your right hip back and under your left hip, stacking your hips. Turn your torso to face the back of your mat, and walk your hands out to lower to your chest. Turn your head to the right, and relax your head to the mat (figure 12.7). Switch sides.

Wheel Pose

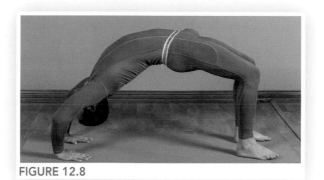

FIGURE 12.8

Wheel pose is perfect for soccer players, because it opens and stretches the whole upper body and creates flexibility in the spine and back. To begin, lie on your mat on your back. Bend both knees, and plant your feet on the mat hip-width apart. Reach both arms up to the ceiling, bend your elbows, and place your palms under your shoulders, fingers pointing to your feet. Lift your hips to the ceiling, and press into your palms to lift your upper body as you relax your neck and drop your head back (figure 12.8).

Frog Pose

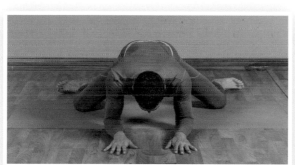

FIGURE 12.9

Frog pose stretches a soccer player's overworked hips and legs. From downward-facing dog pose, lower your knees to the ground to move to your hands and knees. Separate your knees as far apart as possible, keeping your knees in line with your hips. Flexing your feet, line up your ankles with your knees. Lower to your forearms (figure 12.9). Make sure the legs are at a 90-degree angle as you lower to your forearms. Lower to your chest for a deeper stretch.

Summary

This chapter focused on the areas of the body most used on the soccer field. Each pose in the chapter contributes to preventing injuries related to playing soccer. Less-used muscles become tense and stiff, too, so specific poses were added to keep the soccer body balanced.

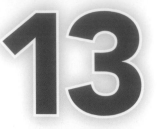

CYCLING: FREE TIGHT HIPS AND A STRESSED UPPER BODY

Cyclists ride for long periods of time, and they need strong, flexible legs and hips to continue the pedaling. Gaining flexibility in these areas that generally get overly tight will allow a cyclist to have a more fluid pedal stroke. Staying flexible in the muscles and loose in the joints will also open more time on the bike during training, allowing for improved performance during competition. It is common for cyclists to experience low-back pain resulting from weak core and back muscles. Yoga offers cyclists core strength and better balance to help with stability on the bike and to prevent pain during races. Another common area of discomfort is the neck and upper back resulting from long periods of leaning forward on the bike. This posture leads to rounded shoulders and a stiff neck from looking forward and up. Yoga opens the front of the body to keep the body balanced and ready for race day. The poses in this chapter address all of these common ailments of bicyclists. Hold each pose for 5 to 10 breaths.

Supported Fish Pose

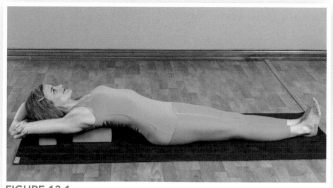

FIGURE 13.1

Cyclists have long training rides and races, so the majority of the time they are leaning forward. Supported fish pose is the counterpose to a cyclist's natural position of being forward for long periods of time. Use two yoga blocks. Place the first block flat at the center of your mat and the second block just behind the first one. Sit in front of the blocks, facing away from them. Slowly lower backward to lie on the first block between your shoulder blades. Rest your head on the second block. Straighten your legs, and bring them together. Reach both arms overhead, and bend your elbows as you clasp the opposite elbow. Relax your forearms down to the floor over your head (figure 13.1). Hold the pose as you breathe. Switch to the opposite forearm on top.

Hips to Wall Pose

A cyclist's repetitive motion on the bike can lead to tightness in the hips. Hips to wall pose targets the muscles cyclists use on the bike to help prolong their rides and increase speed. To begin, lean against a wall. Bend both knees to come into a chair pose against the wall. Place your right ankle on top of your left thigh, keeping your right foot flexed. Lean forward, and place your right elbow to your right arch. Stack your hands, and twist to your left (figure 13.2). As you twist to your left, push your right elbow into your right arch and push your right knee back. Switch sides.

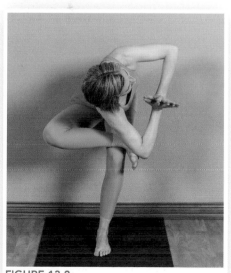

FIGURE 13.2

Wide-Legged Forward Fold

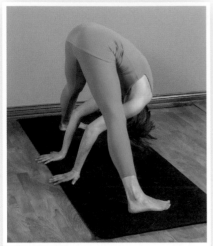

FIGURE 13.3

As a cyclist rides, the push–pull action of pedaling uses the hamstrings a lot. Wide-legged forward fold gives a cyclist the full hamstring stretch needed for riding. From downward-facing dog pose, step your right foot forward between your hands and lift your torso to standing. Turn your right foot to the left so that your feet are parallel to each other. Fold forward, lengthening your head down toward the mat. Turn your hands around and walk the hands back behind you, gripping the mat to lengthen your spine even more (figure 13.3).

Camel Pose

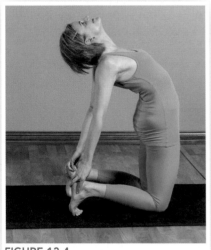

FIGURE 13.4

Long periods of leaning forward on a bike may cause low-back strain. Camel pose allows the rider to stretch the low back and open and stretch the front side body as a counterpose to leaning forward. From downward-facing dog pose, lower your knees to the ground, keeping your toes curled under. Walk your hands back toward your knees, and sit up on your knees. Reach your right hand behind you and take hold of your right heel, then reach your left hand behind you and take hold of your left heel (figure 13.4). Keep your thighs pressing forward, aligning your hips over your knees, and keep your chest lifting as you relax your head back.

Eagle Crunch

Some focus on core work will help a cyclist maintain a strong back and upper torso while on the bike. Eagle crunch helps build this strength. To begin, lie on your back. Bend your knees, and plant both feet on your mat. Cross your right leg over your left leg, wrapping your right foot behind your left ankle. Reach both arms up to the ceiling, and bend your elbows. Hook your right arm under your left arm, wrapping your hands together until your palms or the backs of your hands touch. Lift both legs. Keeping your eagle arms and legs bound, inhale as you reach your fingers overhead and your legs forward (figure 13.5a); exhale as you lift your head and pull your right elbow to your right thigh, tapping them together (figure 13.5b). Repeat this movement 10 to 20 times, then switch sides.

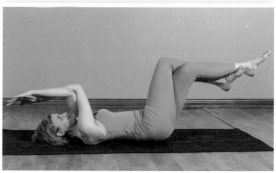
FIGURE 13.5a

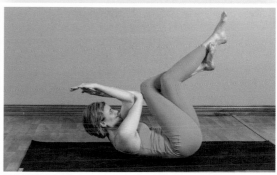
FIGURE 13.5b

Hands and Knees Neck Roll

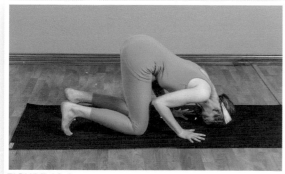
FIGURE 13.6a

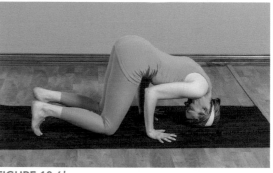
FIGURE 13.6b

Cyclists commonly experience a tight, achy neck from looking forward for long periods of time. Hands and knees neck roll allows the cyclist to easily stretch the neck to keep the muscles relaxed. To begin, come to your hands and knees. Lower your head to the mat, resting at the hairline of your forehead (figure 13.6a). Gently roll over the top of your head until your chin comes to your chest (figure 13.6b). Gently roll back to your hairline. Continue this movement 5 to 10 times.

Eagle Twist

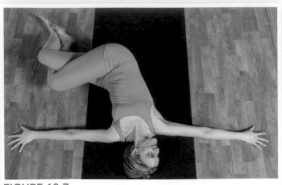

FIGURE 13.7

Cyclists are in the same position for long periods of time. Eagle twist gives your body the stretch and twist it needs after being stationary for a long time. To begin, lie on your back. Reach both arms to your sides, resting your arms to your mat, palms facing down. Bend your knees, and plant both feet on the mat. Cross your right leg over your left leg, and wrap your right foot behind your left ankle. Lift your left foot off the mat, then lower both legs to your left as you look to your right (figure 13.7). Relax, taking deep breaths. Switch sides.

Wall Stretch

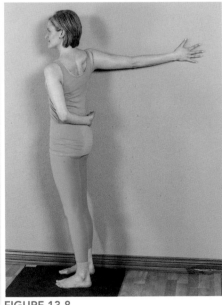

FIGURE 13.8

When on a bike, it's easy to round the shoulders and torso forward. This position leads to shoulder tightness. Wall stretch relieves the shoulders of that tightness and increases the mobility of the shoulders and chest. To begin, stand and face a wall. Place your right palm on the wall at three o'clock. Wrap your left arm behind your back. Turn your feet to the left as you turn your body to the left (figure 13.8). Keep turning until you feel a stretch. Lean into the wall. To come out of the stretch, turn back and face the wall. Place your right hand at two o'clock, and stretch again. For the third round, place your right hand at one o'clock. Repeat the stretch with the left arm.

Half Moon Pose

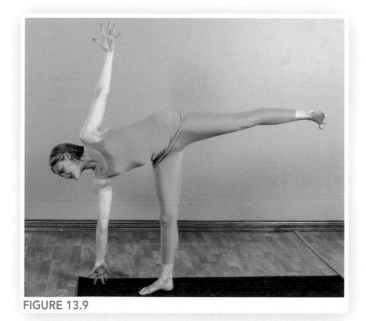

FIGURE 13.9

One may think that cyclists don't need to practice balance postures. However, practicing half moon pose will benefit any cyclist. Balance is especially important to a cyclist, because at a moment's notice something may shoot out in front of you when on the road or you may need to make a quick decision to swerve around debris. Starting from downward-facing dog pose, step your right foot between your hands. Reach your right hand forward, and place your fingertips on the floor. Push off your left foot to balance on your right foot. Flex your left foot, and lift your left leg up to hip height. Stack your hips and your shoulders, reaching your left arm up to the ceiling (figure 13.9). Switch sides.

Twisting High Lunge Pose

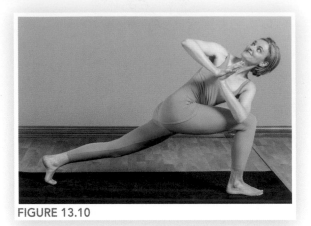

FIGURE 13.10

A cyclist pedals with a push–pull motion. Strong quadriceps muscles increase speed. Twisting high lunge pose gives the quadriceps a deep stretch for relief of muscle soreness and tightness. From downward-facing dog pose, step your right foot forward behind your right hand. Keep your back heel lifted as you lift your torso. Place your left elbow on the outside of your right thigh. Stack your palms in prayer position, and twist to your right (figure 13.10). Switch sides.

Summary

Cyclists need to have not only a strong body but also flexible muscles and joints in order to have the mobility to gain the speed they need for long rides or races. This chapter provided all the key whole-body yoga poses that benefit cyclists so that they can stay on the bike longer, ride faster, and stay injury free.

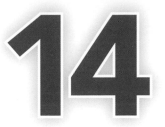

14

BASEBALL AND SOFTBALL: GUARD THOSE JOINTS

Baseball and softball have different positions that require different movements. Flexibility can improve the length of a player's stride while running the bases, shoulder mobility for throwing, acrobatic abilities in the middle infield and outfield, and overall flexibility for first basemen and catchers. Balance can improve agility, leg strength, and focus. All positions need to have the ability to twist when up to bat, but the power comes from the flexibility in the hips. Improving the range of motion in your hips will improve power at the plate. The poses in this chapter will help players in every positon and also keep players balanced and ready for the next game. Hold each pose for 5 to 10 breaths.

Wide-Legged Forward Fold With Strap

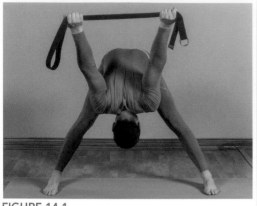

FIGURE 14.1

Every player needs shoulder mobility to throw the ball with precision and velocity. Wide-legged forward fold with strap enhances the ability to maintain mobility and flexibility for a precise throw. From downward-facing dog pose, step your right foot forward between your hands, and lift your torso to standing. Turn your right foot to the left so that your feet are parallel to each other. Hold a yoga strap behind you, one end in each hand. Place your hands about hip-width apart. Fold your torso forward, lengthening your head toward the ground. Lift your arms away from your low back and keep lifting your knuckles to the ceiling (figure 14.1). Switch legs.

Head to Knee Pose

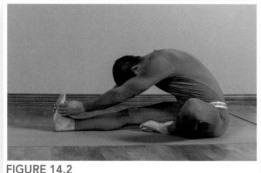

FIGURE 14.2

Sprinting from base to base or racing after a ball requires loose and injury-free hamstrings. Head to knee pose keeps the legs flexible and ready for quick bursts of speed. To begin, sit on your mat. Bend your left knee to your chest, planting the left foot next to the right inner thigh, and lower your left knee to the floor on your left. Flex your right foot as you wrap both hands around your right foot and fold forward (figure 14.2). Switch legs.

Cat/Cow

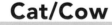

FIGURE 14.3a

Cat/cow gives a player a flexible spine and keeps the back muscles loose for quick, unexpected acrobatic moves on the field. To begin, come to your hands and knees. Inhale as you tilt your head back to look up, lower your belly, and lift your tailbone (figure 14.3a). Exhale as you tuck your chin under, press into your palms, arch your back, and tuck your tailbone (figure 14.3b). Follow your breath with the movement.

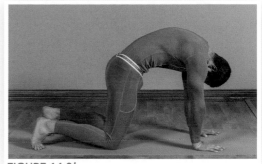
FIGURE 14.3b

One-Legged Frog Pose

Staying balanced in the legs is key for baseball and softball players. One-legged frog pose helps loosen the quadriceps for all positions on the field. From downward-facing dog pose, shift forward to plank pose, then lower to your abdomen. Lift your chest up, aligning your elbows under your shoulders, forearms on the ground. Bend your right knee, and reach your right hand behind you, grabbing your right foot; your fingers face forward. Bend your right elbow to the ceiling as you pull your right foot toward your right hip (figure 14.4). Switch sides.

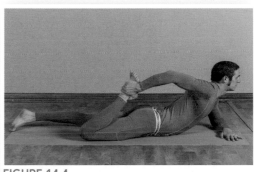
FIGURE 14.4

Lower Core Hip Lift

The many twists, turns, leaps, and other movements needed for baseball and softball require a flexible core. The lower core hip lift will keep the core strong but also protect the back and torso from any strain or pain while on the field. Begin on your back with both knees bending into your chest. Lengthen both arms down along your sides, placing your palms down on the mat. Straighten both legs up to the ceiling, keeping your legs together. Press your low back into the mat, and exhale to lift your hips off the mat (figure 14.5). Inhale to slowly lower your hips. Follow this action with your breath.

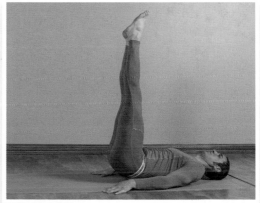
FIGURE 14.5

One-Legged Chair Pose

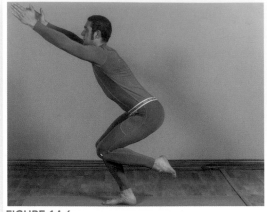

FIGURE 14.6

The uneven ground on the field will challenge all players and all positions. One-legged chair pose strengthens the ankles, feet, and focus to improve balance on the playing field. Stand at the top of your mat with your legs together. Bend your knees, and sit your hips back and down, reaching your arms to the ceiling. Lean to your right, putting all of your weight onto your right foot. Bend your left knee, and pull your left heel up to your left hip (figure 14.6). Switch sides.

Cobra Pose

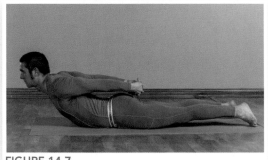

FIGURE 14.7

After all the swinging, running, and squatting in baseball and softball, a backbend is always a refreshing stretch. Cobra pose gives the baseball or softball player the back stretch needed for muscle relief. From downward-facing dog pose, shift forward to a plank pose, lowering your body to the mat. Rest your forehead on the mat. Reach both arms behind you, and interlace your fingers. Press the tops of your feet down into the mat as you lift your head and lengthen your chest forward and up (figure 14.7). Keep your knuckles pressing back as a bound cobra variation.

Happy Baby Pose and Half Happy Baby Pose

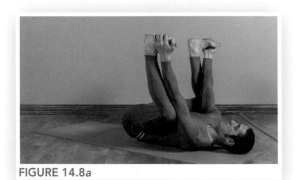

FIGURE 14.8a

Catchers need to have mobile and flexible hips to sit in the squat and explode up to standing for out-of-reach catches or lightning-speed throws to catch a potential base stealer. Happy baby pose and half happy baby pose provide a good hip stretch needed for the field. To begin, lie on your back, pulling both knees in to your chest. Separate your knees, and bring both arms between your knees. Reach your hands over the tops of your ankles, and clasp the outer edges of both feet. Press down to pull your knees toward the mat (figure 14.8a). Release your left foot to the mat, keeping the knee bent (figure 14.8b). Continue to press the right foot down. Switch feet for half happy baby pose on the left leg.

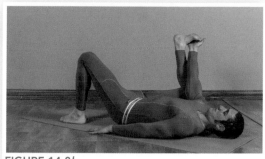
FIGURE 14.8b

Wrist Stretch

After batting or throwing the ball, the hands and wrists need a stretch. Wrist stretch targets exactly the right stretch all players need for the wrists and hands. To begin, come to your hands and knees. Circle your right hand clockwise, planting your palm on the mat so that your fingers point to your right knee. Slowly shift your hips back, keeping your right palm on the floor (figure 14.9). Stop and hold the pose when your feel a stretch in your wrist. Switch wrists.

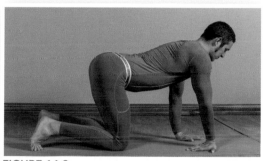
FIGURE 14.9

Seated Spinal Twist

In order to throw the ball, reach high or low, or fall in an unexpected acrobatic motion, a player's torso and spine must have flexibility. Seated spinal twist gives the spine and back muscles the mobility needed for all motions on the field. To begin, sit on your mat with both legs extended in front of you. Bend your left knee to your chest, and place your left foot on the mat on the outside of your right thigh. Bend your right leg, and slide your right foot next to your left hip. Place your left palm on the mat behind your hips. Wrap your right arm around your left knee. Sit tall, and press your left hip down to the mat as you twist to the left (figure 14.10). Switch sides.

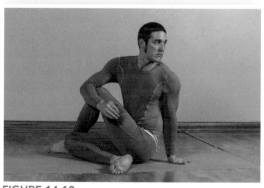
FIGURE 14.10

Eagle Arms

Staying loose in the shoulders is key for baseball and softball players. Eagle arms gives the player the perfect stretch needed for the shoulders. To begin, stand at the top of your mat. Reach both arms out in front of you. Move your right arm under your left arm, and bend both elbows. Wrap your arms around each other so that the palms meet. Press your forearms forward, and lift your fingertips (figure 14.11). Switch the arm on top.

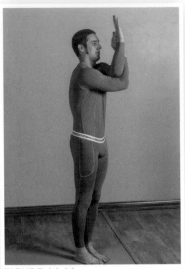

FIGURE 14.11

Open Chest Pose With 90-Degree Arm

All players need to be able to throw the ball; shoulder mobility for a fast pitch or a long throw from the outfield is key. Open chest pose with 90-degree arm is the perfect stretch for baseball and softball players. To begin, lie on your abdomen. Reach your right arm out to your right, and rest the arm on the floor. Bend your right arm, sliding your hand up so that the arm is at a 90-degree angle. Turn your head to look to your left, and rest your head down to the mat. Place your left palm on the mat under your left shoulder. Bend your left knee, and flip your left leg up and over your right leg, resting your left foot on the floor. Press your left palm into the mat, and roll your left shoulder back (figure 14.12). Switch sides.

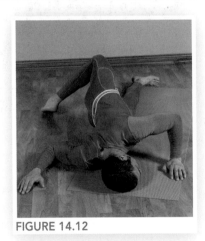

FIGURE 14.12

Summary

Although baseball and softball feature many positions, the poses in this chapter can benefit every player on the field. All players need mobility in the hips and spine for being up to bat. The poses in this chapter benefit players' bodies to enhance playing time on the field.

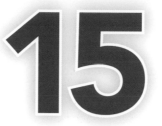

SWIMMING: STRETCH THE SHOULDERS AND BACK

Swimmers build strong shoulders and back muscles, and they need a strong core for twisting as they reach through the water. Injuries tend to be to the shoulders and knees, and swimmers have to do a lot of shoulder and leg stretches to reduce injuries and cramping. Breathing is also important for swimmers to maintain their momentum and rhythm. The poses in this chapter will focus on these areas. The breathing that occurs in every yoga pose will reinforce the rhythmic breathing of swimming. Hold each stretch for 5 to 10 breaths.

Spine Rolling

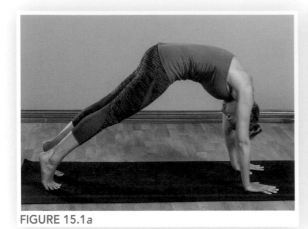

FIGURE 15.1*a*

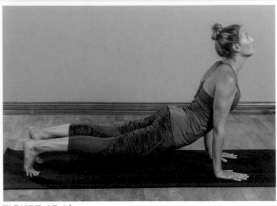

FIGURE 15.1*b*

Full-body mobility and fluid movements are key for swimmers. Spine rolling awakens the whole body before getting into the pool. Starting in downward-facing dog pose, lift both heels high and tuck your chin to your chest. Tuck your tailbone under as you round your whole spine and start to roll forward (figure 15.1*a*). Lower your hips toward the floor as you pull your chest forward and lift your chin up in an upward-facing dog pose (figure 15.1*b*). Then, tuck your chin under and start to round your upper back through your whole back as you return to downward-facing dog pose.

Crisscross Pose

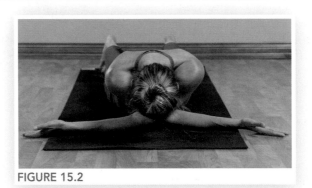

FIGURE 15.2

One of the most used parts of the body and a common site for injury is the shoulders. Crisscross pose provides a shoulder stretch to ease tightness and tension in the shoulders. Lie down on your abdomen, and rest on both forearms. Turn your right palm faceup. Slide your right arm behind your left arm, and straighten your right arm to the left. Then flip your left palm up, and straighten your left arm to the right so that both arms cross each other (figure 15.2). Relax your head down to the floor. Switch the arm on top.

Low Lunge Pose With Block

Keeping the hips loose gives a swimmer power through the legs. Low lunge pose with block gives the swimmer the stretch needed to unleash the power of the legs. From downward-facing dog pose, step your right foot forward, lowering your back knee to the floor to a low lunge. Place a block on the mat on the inside of your right foot. Place both forearms on the block (figure 15.3). Keep your right knee next to your right shoulder as you stay in a low lunge. Keep your spine long, and gaze slightly forward. Switch legs.

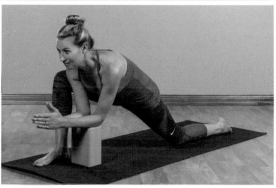

FIGURE 15.3

Revolved Bound Forward Fold

Keeping the hamstrings loose can help prevent cramping and the chances of knee pain or injury. Revolved bound forward fold gives a swimmer the deep hamstring stretch needed in the pool. Stand at the top of your mat, feet hip-width apart. Fold forward, and deeply bend both knees. Take your right shoulder under your right knee. Reach your left arm over and behind you as your right arm reaches under your right leg and you interlace your fingers. Straighten both legs, and turn your left shoulder back (figure 15.4). Switch sides.

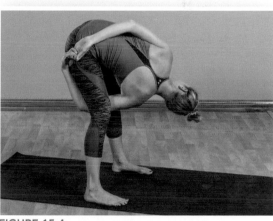

FIGURE 15.4

Low Lunge Pose

Along with the hamstrings, the quadriceps have a large impact on a swimmer for power in the pool and protection of the knees. Lunge pose gives the swimmer the balance of stretching the quadriceps to prevent cramping and injury. From downward-facing dog pose, step your right foot forward between your hands, and lower your left knee to the ground. Place both hands on your right knee, and lift your chest so that your shoulders are above your hips. Bend your right knee, and sink your hips forward and down (figure 15.5). Switch legs.

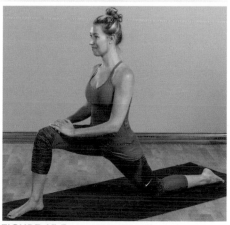

FIGURE 15.5

Dancer Pose

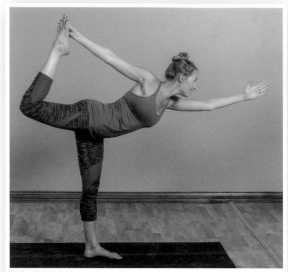

FIGURE 15.6

Swimmers need flexible backs for the various strokes required in the pool. Dancer pose gives a swimmer the deep backbend needed to stay loose and mobile while also working the stabilizers in the standing leg. To begin, stand at the top of your mat. Put your weight on your left foot. Bend your right knee, and with your right hand reach down for the inside of your right foot. Lift your left arm out in front. Push your right foot into your right hand as you lean your upper body forward. As you push your right foot into your hand, lift the foot to the ceiling (figure 15.6). Keep reaching and lengthening forward. Switch legs.

Windshield Wiper Twist

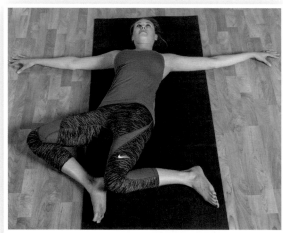

FIGURE 15.7a

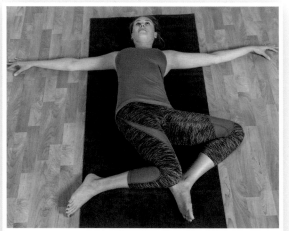

FIGURE 15.7b

Swimmers need strong backs to deal with the repetitive motion of the arms. Windshield wipers is a great stretch for the back muscles and the spine. To begin, lie on your back. Reach both arms out to your sides, and place your palms facedown on the floor. Bend both knees, and plant your feet wider than hip-width apart. Lower both knees to the floor on your right (figure 15.7a). Lift your knees back up, and lower both knees to the floor on your left (figure 15.7b). Keep moving side to side.

Two-Legged Lower and Lift

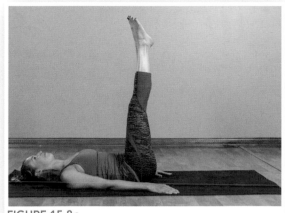

FIGURE 15.8a

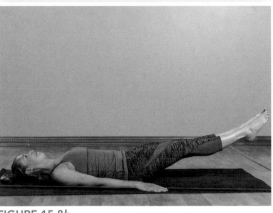

FIGURE 15.8b

A swimmer's core is key in each stroke taken in the pool. The core is the powerhouse that provides the swimmer the strength needed for longer and faster strokes. Two-leg lower and lift helps build a swimmer's core for strong strokes in the pool. To begin, lie on your back. Bend both knees up to your chest, then straighten your legs together to the ceiling (figure 15.8a). Reach your arms down along your sides with your palms down. Press your low back into the floor, and keep your shoulders down away from your ears and pressing into the floor. Lengthen your legs, and slowly lower your legs until they hover above the floor (figure 15.8b). Slowly lift both legs back up. Keep repeating this movement slowly.

Standing Split

Balance is key for everyone, including swimmers. Standing split gives a swimmer the challenge of balancing on one leg while being upside down. To begin, stand at the top of your mat. Put your weight onto your left foot, and lengthen your right leg back. Slowly fold forward, placing your hands on the floor. Walk your hands back to your left foot as you lift your right leg up and fold forward into your left leg (figure 15.9). Switch legs.

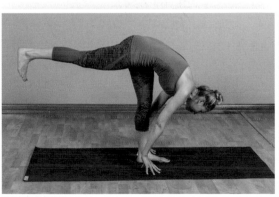

FIGURE 15.9

Summary

Swimmers use the whole body for swimming. This chapter provided poses to help swimmers stay mobile and injury free for competitions. Each pose offers unique stretches to help prevent muscle cramping and fatigue while in the pool. Linking the breath with the pose keeps swimmers focused on poses and breathing simultaneously to prepare for the coordinated movement and breathing required in the pool.

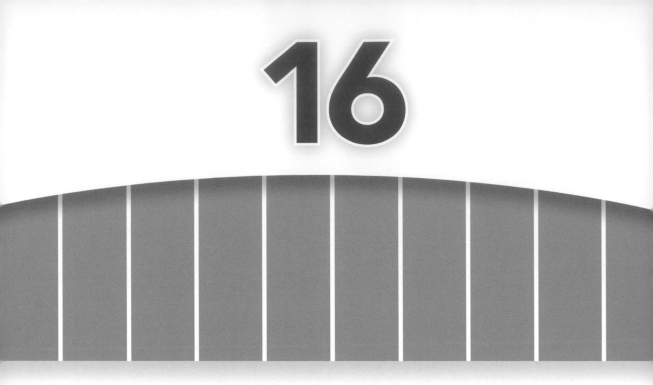

TENNIS: QUICK BURSTS OF MOTION

One of the most important assets a tennis player can have is flexibility. The ability to reach for a ball at any height or angle in a split second on the court is key when competing. A broad range of motion in the dominant shoulder and an arch in the back contribute to power and stability for the serve. All in all, tennis players take a beating from tennis both mentally and physically. For players to prolong their tennis careers, they must maintain a flexible body, relaxed mind, and steady breath. A regular yoga practice provides these tools to enhance performance on the court. The yoga poses in this chapter will help keep the body flexible and mobile for the next match. Hold each pose for 5 to 10 breaths.

Supine Cow Face Legs

Tennis players must be quick on their feet with quick bursts of explosive movements. Supine cow face legs gives a tennis player flexibility in the hips for quick lateral movements. To begin, lie on your back, bend your knees, and plant your feet on the mat. Cross your right leg over your left thigh, stacking your knees. Lift both knees to your chest. With your right hand, reach down for your left foot, then reach down with your left hand for your right foot. Lift both feet up about knee height, and gently pull your feet toward your shoulders (figure 16.1). Switch legs.

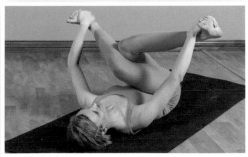
FIGURE 16.1

Revolved Head to Knee Pose

Long, split-second strides are very important during a match. Revolved head to knee pose keeps the hamstrings long and loose for split-second extension of the legs. Sit on your mat with both legs straight in front of you. Separate your legs as wide apart as possible. Bend your left leg, and slide your left foot up to your hips. With your right hand, reach down and clasp your right foot, keeping your right arm on the inside of your right leg. Lift your left arm up and over your head as you lean your torso to your right. With your left hand, clasp your right foot. Roll your left shoulder back and right shoulder forward (figure 16.2). Switch legs.

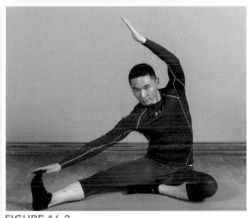
FIGURE 16.2

Twisting Triangle Pose

The backhand is an important part of each tennis player's game. Mobility in the spine and back muscles is key to a powerful, precise backhand. Twisting triangle pose provides the twist needed for the court. From downward-facing dog pose, step your right foot forward behind your right hand. Turn your back heel down, and stand. Square your hips to the front of your mat, and lengthen your spine forward. Plant your left palm on the floor on the outside of your right foot. Keep your hips squared to the front of your mat and your spine long as you twist to your right. Reach your right arm up to the ceiling (figure 16.3). Switch sides.

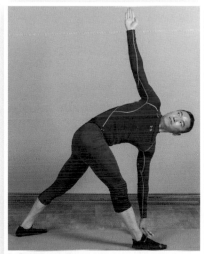
FIGURE 16.3

One-Leg Fingertip Crunch

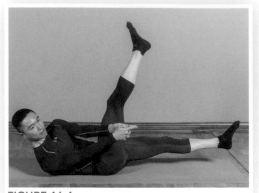

FIGURE 16.4

A strong core is the foundation for a strong body that is likely to stay injury free. One-leg fingertip crunch strengthens the core and improves stability to prevent minor injuries. Lie on your back. Lift your right leg to the ceiling, and hover your left leg off the floor. Reach both arms up and interlace your fingers, leaving your index fingers pointing out. Lift your head and shoulders off the mat, and take your index fingers to the outside of your right leg (figure 16.4). Squeeze your core as you pulse your torso slowly. Switch legs.

Reclining Hero Pose

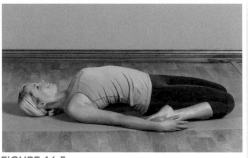

FIGURE 16.5

Staying balanced in the legs is important for tennis play, and keeping the quadriceps healthy and loose is key. Hero pose provides the flexibility needed in the quadriceps while on the court. From downward-facing dog pose, bend both knees and lower to your hands and knees. Uncurl your toes, and place the tops of your feet on the mat. Separate your feet just past hip-width apart. Slowly sit down between your feet, and bring your knees together. Place your hands on the mat behind your hips, and walk yourself down onto your back, keeping your tailbone tucked under. Once you are down onto your back, lengthen your arms down along your sides (figure 16.5).

Eagle Pose

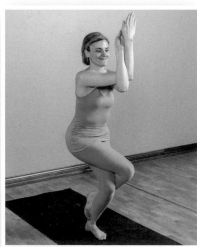

FIGURE 16.6

Unexpected leaps, jumps, and long extensions are common on the tennis court. A balance practice keeps a player ready for unexpected split-second moments. Eagle pose trains the focus of balance needed for the court. To begin, stand at the top of your mat. Bend both knees, and sit your hips back. Put your weight on your left foot, and lift your right leg. Cross your right leg over your left leg. Wrap your right foot behind your left ankle. Reach your arms out in front of you, taking your left arm under your right arm, then bend both elbows, wrapping your arms until your palms meet (figure 16.6). Press your forearms forward, and lift your fingertips. Switch sides.

Cow Face Arms

Shoulder mobility is important for the various angles and height needed for the tennis swing. Cow face arms increases the range of motion needed for all angles of the swing. This pose adds internal and external rotation of the shoulder in one stretch. To begin, stand at the top of your mat. Reach your right arm up overhead toward the ceiling and relax your left arm down along your left side. Bend your left elbow, internally rotating the shoulder, and place the back of your left hand on your low back. At the same time, reach your right arm overhead, externally rotating the shoulder, and bend your right elbow, placing your right hand on your upper back. Slowly slide both hands together, and interlace your fingers (figure 16.7). If your hands don't connect, you can drop a strap from the top arm to the bottom arm to connect them. Switch the top arm.

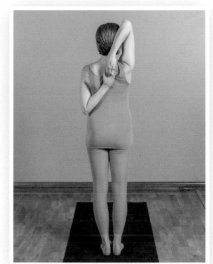

FIGURE 16.7

Wild Thing Pose

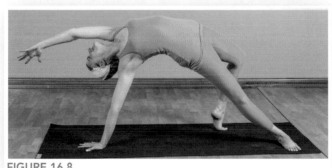

FIGURE 16.8

A powerful serve requires significant spine mobility. Wild thing pose opens the back to increase flexibility of the spine and stretch out the muscles of the back. Starting from downward-facing dog pose, sweep your right leg up high to three-legged downward-facing dog pose. Bend your right knee and externally rotate your hip, lifting your right knee high. Pivoting on the ball of the foot, turn to the outer edge of your left foot. Slowly lower the ball of your right foot to the floor behind your left leg. Lift your hips and chest as you reach your right arm to the front of your mat, and relax your head back (figure 16.8). Switch sides.

Summary

Tennis players need to spring, lunge, leap, or reach for the ball in a split second. Flexibility and balance are important to prepare the body for these actions at a moment's notice. The yoga poses in this chapter prepare a tennis player's body for the next match.

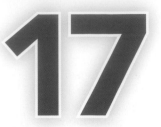

BASKETBALL: EXPLOSIVE MOVEMENT

Basketball is a fast-paced sport that requires balance, body control, constant explosive movement, and high endurance. Basketball players want to move fluidly and stay on the court longer; to ensure success on the court, their joints must have full range of motion. Players also require moments of concentrated mental control on the court; yoga teaches players to be in the moment, listen to their bodies, and focus on breathing. They have to think fast, move fast, respond quickly, and concentrate during times of pressure. All these requirements put special challenges on the body. A regular yoga practice will help to meet these challenges to improve an athlete's recovery time and prevent injury. The poses in this chapter provide a great complement to a basketball player's training. Hold each pose for 5 to 10 breaths.

Wall Stretch

A basketball player's legs are always in motion, and all the muscles of the legs are constantly used. Wall stretch gives a player a deep quadriceps stretch to help prevent injury in the knees and hips. To begin, come to a wall with your mat and two yoga blocks. Place your mat along the wall, then lower to your hands and knees, facing away from the wall. Place the blocks in between your hands on the mat. Lift your right leg, and place your right shin on the wall. Slowly lower your right knee to the floor. Place both hands on the yoga blocks, then lift your left knee and plant your left foot on the mat in a low lunge. Lift your chest, and place both hands on your left thigh (figure 17.1). Slowly move your back and hips to the wall. Switch legs.

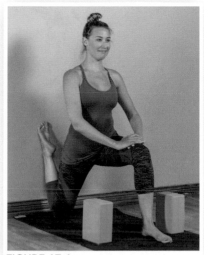

FIGURE 17.1

Crossed Ankles Forward Fold

The constant pounding from running up and down the court will easily tighten the hamstrings. Standing forward fold with legs crossed gives a basketball player the deep hamstring stretch needed for game day. To begin, stand at the top of your mat. Step your right foot in front and to the outside of your left foot. Bend both knees and fold forward, placing your hands on the mat. Straighten both legs, keeping both feet planted on the mat. Walk your hands to the left side of your mat, and hold the position (figure 17.2a). Then walk your hands to the right side of your mat, and hold the position (figure 17.2b). Walk your hands back to your feet, and fold forward. Switch legs.

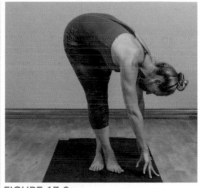

FIGURE 17.2a

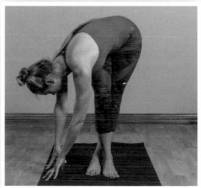

FIGURE 17.2b

Low Lunging Half Pigeon Pose

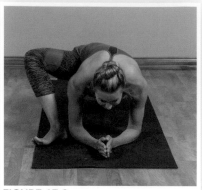

FIGURE 17.3

Basketball requires a lot of lateral movements on the court. Low lunging half pigeon pose provides the flexibility and freedom in the hips to move smoothly and quickly in lateral motions. From downward-facing dog pose, step your right foot forward between your hands and lower your back knee to the mat. Place both hands on the mat on the inside of your right foot. Flex your right toes up, and roll to the outer edge of your right foot, relaxing your right knee as far to the right as is comfortable. Place your forearms on the floor in place of your hands (figure 17.3). Switch legs.

Forward Fold With Shoulder Stretch

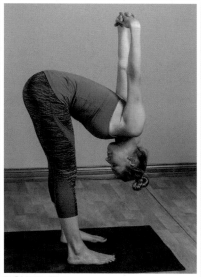

FIGURE 17.4

Having the extension in the arms to block a shot or pass is key for good defense. Standing forward fold with shoulder stretch opens the shoulders for greater mobility for extension on defense or for shooting the ball on offense. To begin, stand at the top of your mat with your feet about hip-width apart. Interlace your fingers behind you. Fold forward and lift your knuckles to the ceiling (figure 17.4).

Warrior III Pose to Jiva Squat

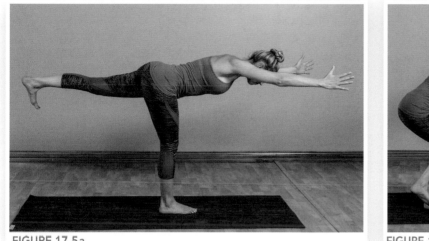

FIGURE 17.5a

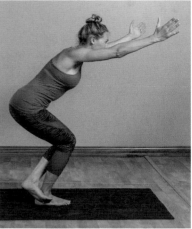

FIGURE 17.5b

At any moment for any position on the basketball court, balance is crucial. A player must maintain proper body control while on the court; often times, body control must be maintained on one foot or in unusual positions. Jiva squat trains a basketball player for moments like these on the court. From downward-facing dog pose, step your right foot forward and lift your torso into warrior III pose (figure 17.5a). Bend both knees. Lower your right knee to a low squat, and bend your left knee to touch your right ankle (figure 17.5b). Slowly lift back up to warrior III, and slowly lower back down, moving with your breath. Switch legs.

Bicycle

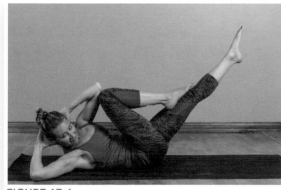

FIGURE 17.6a

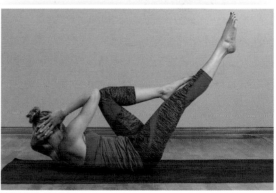

FIGURE 17.6b

Basketball players must be quick and explosive on the court. A strong core gives a player the strength to move quickly. Bicycle is a great way to stay strong in the core. To begin, lie on your back. Place your hands behind your head, keeping your elbows wide, and pull both knees to your chest as you lift your head and shoulders. Inhale as you straighten your right leg. Exhale as you turn to the left, touching your right elbow to your left knee (figure 17.6a). Inhale back to center, straighten your left leg, and pull your right knee back over your hips. Exhaling, twist to your right, and touch your left elbow to your right knee (figure 17.6b). Repeat this movement while coordinating it with your breath.

227

Extended Angle Pose and Twisted Crescent Lunge Pose

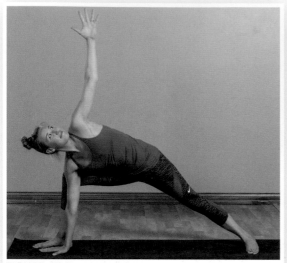

FIGURE 17.7a

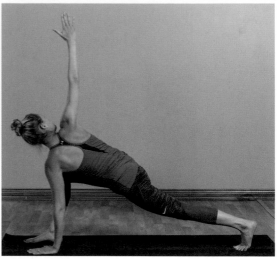

FIGURE 17.7b

Quick twists and turns on the court require a mobile back. Moving between extended angle pose and twisted crescent lunge pose keeps the player's spine and back muscles loose and flexible for those quick twists and turns. To begin, from your downward facing dog, step your right foot forward between your hands and angle your back heel down to the mat. Lift up to standing and bend your right knee forward over your right knee. Reach both arms out of your shoulder as you have come to warrior II pose on the right side. Place your right palm on the mat on the inside of your right foot, and lift your left arm to the ceiling for extended angle pose (figure 17.7a). Place your left palm on the mat next to your right hand. Lifting your left heel off the mat and twisting to your right, reach your right arm to the ceiling (figure 17.7b). Then place your right palm back on the mat on the inside of your right foot. Angle your left heel back to the mat, and reach your left arm up to the ceiling. Keep breathing in coordination with the twisting movement. Switch sides, beginning in warrior II on the left side.

Locust Pose

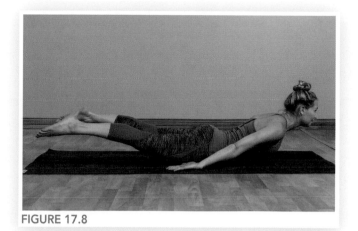

FIGURE 17.8

Basketball players are always in motion and must be ready for the next move on the court. This constant movement leads to a forward lean in the upper body; locust pose is a great backbend for counteracting this forward posture. From downward-facing dog pose, shift forward to plank pose, lowering your abdomen to the ground. Lengthen your arms down along your sides, resting your forehead on the floor. Lift your head, and lengthen your chest forward and up as you lengthen your legs back and lift them off the mat (figure 17.8). Press the back of your hands down onto the mat, keeping your tailbone tucked back to maintain a long body.

Summary

Basketball is a fast-paced sport that requires focus, balance, and body control. The poses in this chapter help basketball players with recovery time and prevent injuries by increasing mobility throughout the whole body. They will allow players to move fluidly and stay on the court longer on game day.

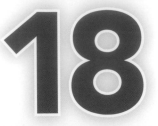

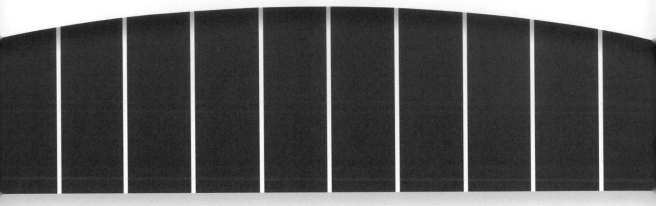

GOLF: LENGTHEN AND ROTATE THE SPINE

Golf isn't just about the swing. A golfer is an athlete, and an athlete trains the whole body. Strength, stamina, balance, stability, mobility, and flexibility are all important for the golf athlete. Incorporating all of these aspects in training will not only help with a strong golf swing, it will keep the body balanced on both sides. Yoga poses increase the range of motion around the joints and the elasticity of the muscles or muscle groups to lengthen and loosen tight areas. When these areas are mobile and flexible, muscles will move faster and more fluidly, increasing power and accuracy in the golfer's game. Hold each pose for 5 to 10 breaths.

Eye of the Needle Pose

The power of the swing doesn't come from the arms; it comes from the lower body. Eye of the needle pose opens the hips so that they can produce the power needed for the drive. To begin, lie on your back. Bend both knees, and plant your feet on the mat about hip-width apart. Lift your right leg, then place your right ankle on your left quadriceps, keeping your right foot flexed. Lift your left foot off the mat, and wrap both hands around your left thigh. Gently pull your left knee toward your chest (figure 18.1). Switch legs.

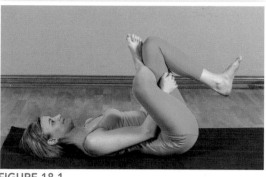

FIGURE 18.1

Supine Big Toe Hold

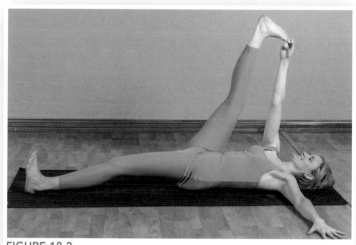

FIGURE 18.2

Golfers walk a lot, bend down, and lean over for the ball while in a match. Staying loose in the hamstrings keeps the back of the body open and free of pain. Supine big toe hold gives the golfer the target stretch needed to stay loose. To begin, lie on your back. Pull your right knee to your chest, and lengthen your left leg to your mat. Wrap the index and middle fingers of your right hand around your right big toe. Straighten your right leg up to the ceiling, pushing up through your right heel and flexing your toes down (figure 18.2). Gently pull your right leg toward your chest, keeping your leg straight. Switch legs.

Twisting Chair Pose

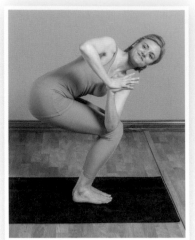

FIGURE 18.3

Keeping the spine and back muscles loose, flexible, and balanced adds to the quality of a golfer's swing. Twisting chair pose is a key pose for the mobility of the back muscles and spine. To begin, stand at the top of your mat. Bend both knees, taking your hips back and down as you lift your chest and arms up to a chair pose. Bring your palms together and down to your chest. Place your left elbow to the outside of your right knee. Press your right palm into your left palm as you twist to your right (figure 18.3). Return to chair pose, then twist to your left.

Sliding Knee Tuck

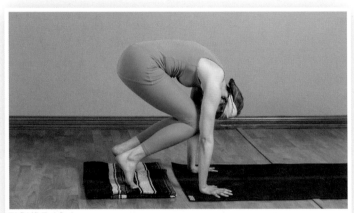

FIGURE 18.4

A strong core not only helps with a golf swing, it also keeps the back strong and injury free. Sliding knee tuck provides the core strength needed for power in the swing and protection of the back from injury. Start in a plank pose with your palms on the end of your mat and your feet on a blanket on a slippery floor. On your exhale, bend both knees, and pull your knees to your chest, tucking your chin under (figure 18.4). Inhale and lengthen your whole body back to plank pose. Repeat this motion for 10 to 15 reps for 2 to 3 sets.

Warrior III Pose

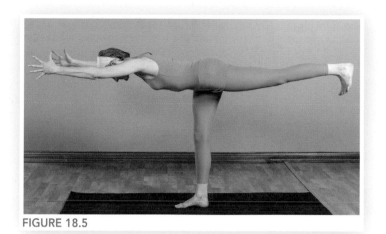

FIGURE 18.5

Walking on uneven ground while on the course requires balance. The steadiness and preciseness of a swing or putt also requires balance. Warrior III pose trains the steadiness and balance needed for the course. Start from downward-facing dog pose. Step your right foot forward between your hands. Push off your back foot, lifting it to hip height, and balance on your right leg. Reach both arms overhead, pushing back through your left heel (figure 18.5). Switch legs.

Sphinx Pose

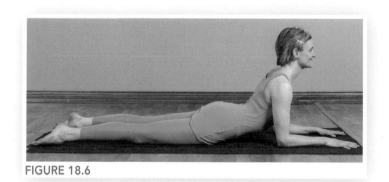

FIGURE 18.6

A golf game requires a golfer to slightly lean forward for the swing or putt. Reversing this action with sphinx pose stretches out the upper and middle back muscles and spine. From downward-facing dog pose, shift forward to plank pose and lower to your abdomen. Lift up to your forearms, aligning your elbows under your shoulders, palms flat and fingers pointing to the top of your mat. Press the tops of your feet into the mat to engage your thighs. Tuck your tailbone toward your heels. Press your palms down into the mat, and slightly pull the ground back, allowing you to push your chest forward and up, keeping your shoulders back (figure 18.6).

Twisting Low Lunge Pose

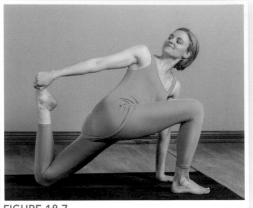

FIGURE 18.7

Staying balanced in the legs is key with the amount of walking, squatting, and swinging done in a match. Twisting low lunge pose gives a golfer a great quadriceps stretch needed for all the movements needed for the course. From downward-facing dog pose, step your right foot forward between your hands and lower your left knee to the mat in a low lunge. Lift your chest, and place both hands on your right thigh as you sink into a low lunge. Reach back with your right hand, and grab your left foot. Place your left palm on the floor on the inside of your right foot. Turn your right shoulder to the right, looking behind you (figure 18.7). Sink deeper into the low lunge. Switch sides.

Supine Half Cow Face Arms

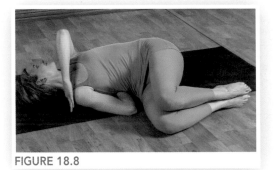

FIGURE 18.8

When a golfer repeatedly leans forward to take a full swing or putt, eventually tightness in the shoulders results. Supine half cow face arms gives the golfer the exact stretch needed for a better range of motion for the swing. To begin, lie on your back. Bend your knees, and plant your feet on the mat. Lift your right hip off the mat and slide your right hand under your low back with the palm on the mat. Lower your right hip to your hand. Pull both knees up to your chest, and lower both knees to the floor on your right. Cross your left arm over your chest, and touch the ground on the right side of your mat (figure 18.8). Switch sides.

Summary

The golf swing is not only in the arms; it involves the whole body. A golfer needs to have a balanced body and loose muscles and joints to stay injury free and maintain a precise swing or putting stroke. Each of the poses in this chapter increases flexibility and mobility to help balance the golfer's body, setting it up for success on the course.

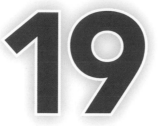

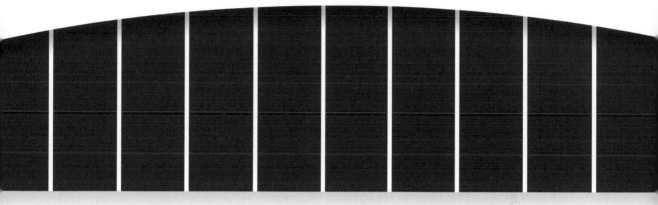

HIGH-INTENSITY TRAINING: FUNCTION AND POWER

The human body is strong and is capable of being pushed much further than one can imagine. To push the body further, you must allow extra time for recovery. To squat deeper or to improve a clean or snatch, you need to have full range of motion and mobility in the hips and shoulders. Lifting does increase strength, but yoga can add to that strength by introducing the body to new movements. Strength is gained through balance postures and slow movements from one pose to the next. Moving fast in yoga isn't always better. Yoga and power workouts go hand in hand, because both require proper breathing techniques and a focal point in practice. Yoga will increase the focus and control required by power workouts to achieve personal goals. Hold each pose for 5 to 10 breaths.

Thread the Needle Pose

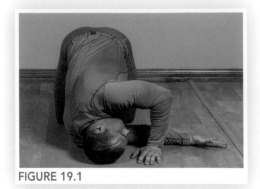

FIGURE 19.1

The shoulders take on a lot, and shoulder mobility is key to freeing the shoulders. To have the full range of motion in an overhead press, thread the needle pose helps to open the shoulders for a better lift. From downward-facing dog pose, bend both knees and lower to your hands and knees. Put your weight onto your left palm, and slide your right arm to the left between your left arm and left leg with your right palm faceup. Lower your right shoulder and right ear to the mat. Press your left palm down into the mat, twisting your left shoulder back (figure 19.1). Switch sides.

Seated Wide-Legged Forward Fold

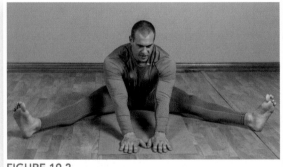

FIGURE 19.2

Even when technique is correct, strength building creates tightness. For example, properly doing deadlifts strengthens the hamstrings but can cause tightness in the same muscles. Seated wide-legged forward fold stretches the hamstrings to keep them loose. To begin, sit on your mat. Separate your legs as wide apart as possible. Place your hands on the mat in front of your hips. Walk your hands forward as you lean your torso toward the ground (figure 19.2).

Supine Spinal Twist

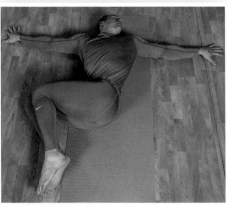

FIGURE 19.3

Power workouts do not feature many movements that require twisting, so adding supine spinal twist provides spinal flexibility and muscle flexibility needed to stay loose. To begin, lie on your mat with both knees bent up to your chest; your arms are reaching out wide with the palms facedown. Slowly lower your legs to the right toward the floor as you look to the left (figure 19.3). Switch sides.

Crescent Lunge Pose

Front squats strengthen the quadriceps, but they can also tighten them. Crescent lunge pose provides a deep stretch needed in the quadriceps. From downward-facing dog pose, step your right foot forward behind your right hand. Keep your left heel up as you lift your torso and reach your arms overhead. Bend your right knee forward, and at the same time push back through your left heel (figure 19.4). Keep your tailbone tucking under and your core slightly engaged. Switch legs.

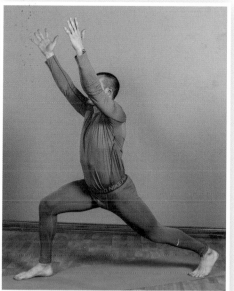

FIGURE 19.4

Plank Pose With Heels Side to Side

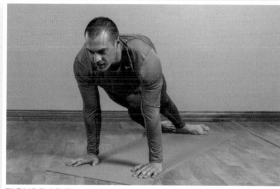

FIGURE 19.5a

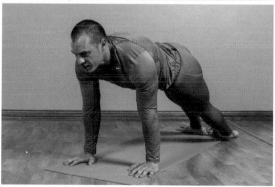

FIGURE 19.5b

Core work is not a favorite for many people, but staying strong in the core protects the torso from injury and will aid in lifting. Plank heels side to side targets the muscles needed for lifting. From downward-facing dog, shift forward to high plank pose. Separate your feet about hip-width apart. Stay stable in the upper body, and engage your core. Exhale and roll both heels to the right toward the ground (figure 19.5a). Inhale and lift your heels back up, and exhale and roll them to the left down to the ground (figure 19.5b). Repeat this movement with the breath for 10 to 15 reps for 2 to 3 sets.

Tree Pose

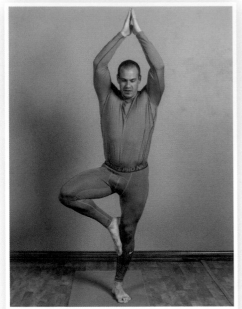

FIGURE 19.6

Balance is important for any lift. Good balance promotes joint stability of the knees, hips, ankles, and shoulders to prevent a whole array of injuries. Tree pose helps train the balance needed for any lift by promoting body awareness. Stand on your mat. Put your weight on your left foot. Bend and lift your right knee up. Turn your right knee to the right, and place your right foot on your inner left thigh. Reach both arms up over your head with your palms together (figure 19.6). Switch legs.

Upward-Facing Dog Pose

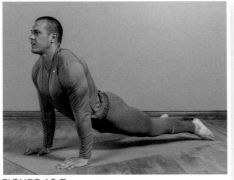

FIGURE 19.7

Bending down to pick up weights or performing back strengthening workouts demands a lot of work from the back muscles. Upward-facing dog pose stretches all the muscles of the back to ease tightness and to open the back. It also stretches the front side of the body. From downward-facing dog pose, shift forward to plank pose, moving down to your abdomen on the ground. Uncurl your back toes, and place the tops of your feet on the mat. Slide your hands back slightly next to your rib cage. Keep your elbows pressing toward each other as you pull your chest forward. Press your palms into the mat, and lengthen your spine upward as you straighten your arms (figure 19.7). Press the tops of your feet down into the mat, and lift your hips and thighs.

Wide Squat Pose

A lifter always wants to squat deeper without restriction from tightness. Wide squat pose provides a good stretch for a deep, effortless squat. From downward-facing dog pose, step your right foot forward and stand. Turn your right foot to the left, and face the left side of the mat. Slightly turn your heels in and toes out. Bend both knees, and place your hands on the mat. Walk your hands back so that you can place your elbows to your inner thighs. Sink your hips, lift your chest, and push your knees apart (figure 19.8).

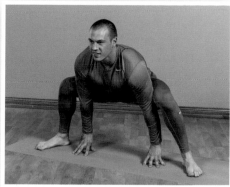

FIGURE 19.8

Summary

Powerlifters are strong and push their bodies to the max. While building the strength in the muscles, flexibility and mobility easily get put aside. This lack of flexibility and mobility leads to injury or a loss of range of motion. All the poses in this chapter give the lifter the mobility and flexibility for a deeper squat or a smoother snatch to increase control and body awareness.

ABOUT THE AUTHOR

Ryanne Cunningham, RYT 200, RYT 500, is a longtime resident of the Green Bay area. She operates Flow Yoga Studio, where she trains current and former Green Bay Packers football players Randall Cobb, Tramon Williams, B.J. Raji, Jarrett Bush, Mike Neal, Andy Mulumba, and others as well as athletes from many other sports in both group and private yoga sessions. Cunningham obtained her 500-hour RYT Advanced Teacher Training certification in 2012 through a yoga center in Green Bay, where she has practiced and taught since 2002. She earned her 200-hour RYT in 2002 at Satchidananda Ashram 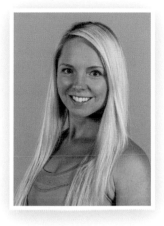 in Buckingham, Virginia, and holds a Power Yoga for Sports certification.

Since 2002 Cunningham has owned and operated Advanced Massage Therapy. Her education in massage therapy covered topics such as human anatomy, biology, and kinesiology, which she uses in her yoga teachings and practices. She uses her personal experience in sports and fitness in teaching students proper stretching and alignment, which benefit all yoga students.

Cunningham has been featured in numerous national and local publications, including *Yoga Journal*, the *Milwaukee Journal Sentinel*, and *Mantra Magazine*.

Find other outstanding fitness resources at

www.HumanKinetics.com/fitness-and-health

In the **U.S.** call 1-800-747-4457
Australia 08 8372 0999
Canada 1-800-465-7301
Europe +44 (0) 113 255 5665
New Zealand 0800 222 062

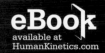

eBook
available at
HumanKinetics.com

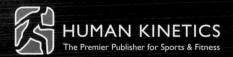

HUMAN KINETICS
The Premier Publisher for Sports & Fitness